OCCASIONAL PUBLICATION NO. 12

VIOLENCE AGAINST WOMEN:

The Health Sector Responds

Marijke Velzeboer
Mary Ellsberg
Carmen Clavel Arcas
Claudia García-Moreno

Produced in collaboration with

PROGRAM FOR APPROPRIATE TECHNOLOGY IN HEALTH

NORWEGIAN AGENCY FOR INTERNATIONAL DEVELOPMENT

SWEDISH INTERNATIONAL DEVELOPMENT AGENCY

PAN AMERICAN HEALTH ORGANIZATION
Pan American Sanitary Bureau, Regional Office of the
WORLD HEALTH ORGANIZATION
525 Twenty-third Street, N.W. Washington, D.C. 20037 U.S.A.

2003

PAHO Library Cataloguing-in-Publication Data

Velzeboer, Marijke
    Violence against women: the health sector responds
Washington, D.C.: PAHO, 2003.
(Occasional Publication No. 12)
ISBN 92 75 12292 X

I. Title   II. Series
III. Ellsberg, Mary   IV. Clavel Arcas, Carmen

1. VIOLENCE AGAINST WOMEN
2. WOMAN
3. GENDER
4. COMMUNITY PARTICIPATION
5. EMPOWERMENT
LC HQ5528.P187 2003

COVER ILLUSTRATION BY LILIANA GUTIÉRREZ
Lápiz y Papel
Quito, Ecuador

DESIGN BY ULTRADESIGNS
Silver Spring, Maryland, U.S.A.

CONTENTS

THE AUTHORS

Marijke Velzeboer, Coordinator for the Women, Health, and Development Program of the Pan American Health Organization (PAHO), prepared Section I (Chapters One through Three). *Mary Ellsberg*, Senior Program Officer, Program for Appropriate Technology in Health (PATH), and *Carmen Clavel Arcas*, International Fellow, National Center for Injury Prevention and Control, U.S. Centers for Disease Control and Prevention (CDC), prepared Section II (Chapters Four through Seven). *Claudia García-Moreno*, Coordinator, Department of Gender and Women's Health of the World Health Organization (WHO) provided the global insights presented in Chapter Eight. *Roberta Okey*, of PAHO Publications, served as the book's editor.

ACKNOWLEDGMENTS

The authors would like to acknowledge the valuable contributions and support of the following individuals, teams, and institutions: PAHO's Janete da Silva and Cathy Cuellar; PATH's Colleen Conroy, Willow Gerber, and Rebeca Quiroga; and CDC's James A. Mercy, Associate Director for Science, Division of Violence Prevention, National Center for Injury Prevention and Control, and Mark Anderson, Division of Emergency and Environmental Health Services, National Center for Environmental Health, for reviewing and commenting on the manuscript drafts. PAHO's Hillary Anderson and PATH's Rebecca Quiroga composed the Resources Section found at the end of the book, and Edna Quirós of PAHO provided administrative support. PAHO's Central American country offices and the Women, Health, and Development Program's network of focal points facilitated the "Lessons Learned" evaluation on which the book is based.

Moreover, the PAHO focal points and their national counterparts in the respective ministries of health, offices of women's affairs, and women's nongovernmental organizations, under the direction of the PAHO Subregional Coordinating team, have been instrumental in developing and implementing the integrated approach to gender-based violence described in the book and in contributing to its achievements. These include the team's current Coordinator, Cathy Cuellar, and her predecessor, Lea Guido, with the assistance of Marta Castillo; focal points Sandra Jones, Belize; Florencia Castellanos, Costa Rica; Amalia Ayala and Ruth Manzano, El Salvador; Elsy Camey, Paula del Cid, Rebeca Guizar, and Patricia Ruiz, Guatemala; Raquel Fernández, Honduras; Silvia Narváez, Nicaragua; and Dora Arosemena, Panama. Janete da Silva provided key support to the Central American network. We also wish to thank the women, men, health care providers, community activists, and representatives of the ministries of health and PAHO for sharing their time, experiences, and knowledge with PAHO and the project evaluation team in a critical, yet constructive spirit.

Clearly, the long-term support of the Governments of Norway and Sweden has not only enabled the development of the integrated approach, the Central American project, and its subsequent evaluation, but the production of this book, as well. Special thanks are due to Carola Espinoza and Mette Kottman and of the Norwegian Agency for International Development (NORAD) and Hans Åkesson of the Swedish International Development Agency (Sida), in particular, for their assistance throughout the project's assessment phase. Likewise, the authors owe a debt of gratitude to the Government of the Netherlands for supporting the contributions of our Bolivian, Ecuadorian, and Peruvian colleagues to this book.

The authors wish to dedicate this book to all the survivors of violence who so courageously have shared their stories with the desire that others might benefit from their experiences and live safer and happier lives. Their situations are both unique and universal, contributing to our knowledge and understanding of gender-based violence and informing our resolve and actions to overcome it. We hope that the lessons learned in Central America will transcend national and cultural boundaries to find resonance everywhere in the world where dedicated and concerned individuals are looking for guidance in making their communities healthier and violence-free.

PREFACE

I am pleased that the publication of this book takes place at the beginning of the Pan American Health Organization's first administration to be headed by a woman, and that in this, my first book preface, I have the opportunity to place on record my commitment to turning the tide against gender-based violence in the Region of the Americas.

The voices of the women you will hear throughout this book's narrative are rooted in the reality of their everyday lives and call for a compassionate response in the form of recognition and an end to their suffering. The first call for action, to be sure, focuses on the health sector. But implicit in the ultimate, all-encompassing response is action by a diverse partnership involving governments and communities of doctors, nurses, and other health professionals working alongside their counterparts: political leaders, the police and court systems, NGOs, schools, and churches.

PAHO's work in Central America to end violence and to utilize health as a bridge to create long-lasting peace began in 1985, and improving the health situation of women was, and continues to be, a cornerstone of the efforts of PAHO and the international community to consolidate democracy and subregional integration. For more than a decade, the Governments of Norway and Sweden have recognized the pivotal role of women in families and communities in the construction of peace at its most basic and elemental level, and the Nordic cooperation's steadfast belief in this principle is largely responsible for the groundwork that has made this book possible.

Finally, I would like this book full of voices to serve as our social conscience as we embark on an international, interagency campaign during 2003 and beyond to lead and support community initiatives to prevent gender-based violence and to empower women and girls everywhere to realize their full potential and offer our societies the rewards of their wisdom and experience.

MIRTA ROSES PERIAGO
Director

INTRODUCTION

Gender-based violence (GBV) is one of the most widespread human rights abuses and public health problems in the world today, affecting as many as one out of every three women. It is also an extreme manifestation of gender inequity, targeting women and girls because of their subordinate social status in society. The consequences of GBV are often devastating and long-term, affecting women's and girls' physical health and mental well-being. At the same time, its ripple effects compromise the social development of other children in the household, the family as a unit, the communities where the individuals live, and society as a whole.

Violence against Women: The Health Sector Responds provides a strategy for addressing this complex problem and concrete approaches for carrying it out, not only for those on the front lines attending to the women who live with violence, but also for decision-makers who may incorporate the lessons in the development of policies and resources. For those communities where support for women does not yet exist, the authors hope that this book will motivate health providers and leaders to more directly confront the issue of gender-related violence and ensure support to affected women in resolving their situation.

This book is a collaborative effort between the Pan American Health Organization (PAHO) and the Program for Appropriate Technology in Health (PATH), with technical assistance provided by the U.S. Centers for Disease Control and Prevention (CDC). PAHO produced the first three chapters of Section I: Chapter One gives an overview of why gender-based violence is a public health problem. Chapters Two and Three discuss the development, implementation, and achievements of PAHO's integrated strategy for addressing GBV, starting with how the "Critical Path" study helped define the strategy. In the next four chapters of Section II, PATH presents the strategy's application and its "Lessons Learned" at the macro, or political, level (Chapter Four), within the health sector (Chapter Five), in the clinic (Chapter Six), and beyond the clinic to the community at large (Chapter Seven). The World Health Organization contributed the final chapter (Chapter Eight), which offers a more global perspective on how the lessons learned and the integrated strategy may be applied in other communities around the world.

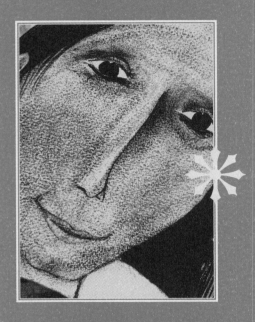

The obstacles to overcoming
family violence are 500
years of culture ingrained
through socialization in
our children.
                    —*Montserrat Sagot, 2001*

SECTION I

The Health Sector Responds to Gender-Based Violence

INTRODUCTION

One important achievement of the last decade is that violence against women is increasingly recognized as a major public health problem. Due in large part to the tireless advocacy of women's organizations, the issue has been placed on the agenda of a number of international conferences: the World Conference on Human Rights (Vienna, 1993), the International Conference on Population and Development (Cairo, 1994), and the Fourth World Conference on Women (Beijing, 1995). The commitments made during these conferences by participating governments, international agencies, and donors directed growing attention to this globally alarming problem.

The Convention on the Elimination of All Forms of Discrimination against Women (CEDAW, 1979) and the Inter-American Convention on the Prevention, Punishment, and Eradication of Violence against Women (Belém do Pará, 1994), provide a concrete political framework for action, by calling on governments to develop and monitor legislation and other related actions. Almost all countries in the Region of the Americas have since ratified these conventions and passed legislation penalizing violence against women.

Yet even prior to the existence of international sanctions against GBV, women's organizations in many parts of the Americas had proposed and lobbied for legislation, formed national coalitions, obtained funding to train police and judges, and provided counseling and services for affected women. The health sector, however, had been conspicuously absent in most of these efforts.

Section I of this book describes PAHO's efforts to mobilize the health sector in joining these forces. Recognizing the pivotal role this sector could play in GBV prevention, in 1993 the Organization passed a resolution calling on its member countries to develop policies and plans for the prevention and management of violence against women.

PAHO's Women, Health, and Development Program was entrusted with developing a health strategy in accordance with the resolution. The following year, the Program and its health sector and other counterparts launched an integrated approach that built upon existing efforts, while strengthening the health sector's participation and contribution in addressing GBV at the policy, service delivery, and community levels. By the end of 2002, a total of 16 countries had implemented this approach; 10 countries with the support of PAHO, and six with the support of the Inter-American Development Bank. The Governments of Sweden and Norway funded PAHO's work in the Central American countries, while the Government of the Netherlands supported work in Bolivia, Ecuador, and Peru.

". . . so I felt that my life had changed, that I was another person, that I was not the same, that I would not suffer anymore. . . . "

—Guatemalan woman

Achievements related to the approach are numerous, but the most significant was the new role of the health sector in joining forces for advocacy, in organizing community networks, and in preventing, detecting, and caring for women and families living with violence. The intersectoral community networks piloted by the new project were subsequently replicated far beyond the initial two networks programmed for each country. Countries shared materials and experiences for training health workers, on developing protocols and information systems, and on starting self-help groups. These experiences leveraged additional support from governments, civil society, and other sources, that in turn resulted in the training of thousands of providers from the health and other sectors, in improved health policies, and in the strengthening of coalitions that advocate for new or better national legislation.

During the implementation period, PAHO's network of focal points for the 10 project countries and their health sector counterparts met yearly to evaluate the project's activities and agree on annual operational plans. While these evaluations revealed a great number of operational achievements, PAHO wanted to know if the project had in reality made a difference in the practices and attitudes of decision-makers, service providers, and the women themselves. Thus, the Women, Health, and Development Program approached its Nordic donors to carry out a participative assessment in the Central America countries.

The donors agreed, and contacted the Program for Appropriate Technology in Health (PATH) and the U.S. Centers for Disease Control and Prevention (CDC) to work with PAHO to carry out the assessment. Both organizations have extensive experience working in Central America on GBV issues and with PAHO, and were thus familiar with the project. The assessment was carried out during October and November, 2001, and included an extensive review of project documents and visits to two selected project sites each in El Salvador, Guatemala, Honduras, and Nicaragua. In Belize, Costa Rica, and Panama, the assessment team interviewed decision-makers and project coordinators from PAHO and the health sector.

The resulting "Lessons Learned" (Ellsberg and Clavel Arcas 2001), attest to the achievements of the project and accredit these to the integrated approach that was applied at all levels, through coalitions, capacity-building of the health and other sectors, and community networks. They also point out the challenges that remain for the health sector in addressing the complex problem of GBV and in its collaboration with other sectors. These "Lessons" provide the basis for this book.

Chapter One

Gender-Based Violence:
A Public Health and Human Rights Problem

Gender-based violence, or "violence against women," includes many kinds of harmful physical, emotional, and sexual behaviors against women and girls that are most often carried out by family members, but also at times by strangers. The United Nations Declaration on the Elimination of Violence against Women includes a widely accepted definition of violence against women as:

> . . . any act of gender-based violence that results in, or is likely to result in, physical, sexual, or psychological harm or suffering to women, including threats of such acts, coercion, or arbitrary deprivations of liberty, whether occurring in public or private life.
> —United Nations General Assembly, 1993

This definition places violence against women within the context of gender inequity as acts that women suffer because of their subordinate social status with regard to men.

There is much debate about a universally agreed-upon GBV terminology. In Latin American countries most laws and policies use the term "family violence" when referring mostly to violence against women by an intimate partner. PAHO initially used the term "family violence" in the early days of its work in this area, but has since shifted to the use of "gender-based violence" or "violence against women" to refer to the broader range of acts that women and girls commonly suffer from intimate partners and family members, as well as individuals outside the family. Thus, both these terms will be used interchangeably throughout the book. The term "family violence" will only be used when referring to the titles of formal laws or programs.

GENDER-BASED VIOLENCE: HOW PREVALENT? HOW COMPLEX?

According to a recent review of 50 studies from around the world, between 10% to 50% of women have experienced some act of physical violence by an intimate partner at some point in their lives (Heise, Ellsberg, and Gottemoeller 1999). This and an earlier World Bank review (Heise, Pitanguy, and Germain 1994) highlight some of the characteristics that often accompany violence in intimate relationships:

➙ The great majority of perpetrators of violence are men; women are at the greatest risk from men they know.

➙ Physical violence is almost always accompanied by psychological abuse and in many cases by sexual abuse.

➙ Most women who suffer any physical aggression by a partner generally experience multiple acts over time.

➙ Violence against women cuts across socioeconomic class and religious and ethnic lines.

➙ Men who batter their partners exhibit profound controlling behavior.

> In León, Nicaragua, among 188 women who were physically abused by their partners, only five were not abused sexually, psychologically, or both.
>
> *—Ellsberg et al. 2000*

These studies show that gender-based violence is a complex problem that can not be attributed to a single cause. There are risk factors, such as alcohol and drug abuse, poverty, and childhood witnessing of or experiencing violence, that contribute to the incidence and severity of violence against women. Overall, however, it is a multicausal problem, influenced by social, economic, psychological, legal, cultural, and biological factors, as illustrated in the figure below.

FIGURE 1-1. ECOLOGICAL MODEL OF FACTORS ASSOCIATED WITH INTIMATE PARTNER VIOLENCE

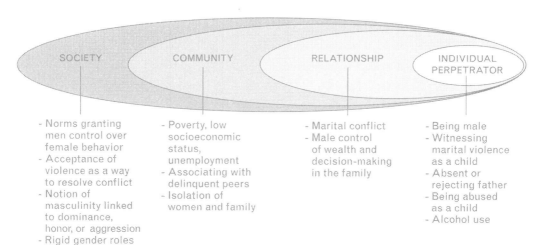

From: Heise, Ellsberg, and Gottemoeller 1999

WHY IS GENDER-BASED VIOLENCE A HEALTH PROBLEM?

As time goes on, there is increasing evidence and awareness among health providers and policymakers of the negative health outcomes of gender-based violence. It has been associated with reproductive health risks and problems, chronic ailments, psychological consequences, injury, and death (Figure 1-2.).

FIGURE 1-2. **HEALTH OUTCOMES OF VIOLENCE AGAINST WOMEN**

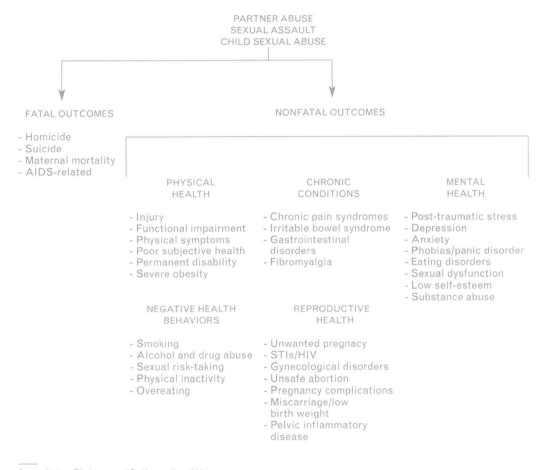

From: Heise, Ellsberg, and Gottemoeller 1999

Physical and sexual abuse affect women's reproductive health, either directly through the risks incurred by forced sex or fear, or indirectly through the psychological effects that lead to risk-taking behaviors. Children may also suffer the consequences, either during the mother's pregnancy, or during their own childhood due to neglect or the psychological and developmental effects of living with or experiencing abuse (Heise, Ellsberg, and Gottemoeller 1999). The following table summarizes how violence undermines women's control over their own reproductive health, as well as the health of their children.

TABLE 1-1. REPRODUCTIVE HEALTH RISKS AND CONSEQUENCES OF VIOLENCE AGAINST WOMEN

- Men who are physically abusive are also more likely to have multiple sexual partners, and to coerce their partners into sex, thereby exposing them to sexually transmitted infections (STI), including HIV.
- Women in abusive relationships are less able to refuse forced sex, use contraception, or negotiate condom use, thereby increasing their risk of unwanted pregnancies and STI/HIV.
- Sexual and physical violence increase women's risk for many reproductive health problems, such as chronic pelvic pain, vaginal discharge, sexual dysfunction, and premenstrual problems, as well as pregnancy loss from abortion or miscarriage, and low birthweight in infants.
- Fear, geographical isolation, and lack of economic resources may prevent women from seeking reproductive health services—prenatal care, gynecological and contraceptive services, STI/HIV screening and care—and to adequately care for their children.
- Witnessing or experiencing violence against women during childhood has been associated with risk-taking behavior during adolescence and adulthood: early sexual initiation, adolescent pregnancy, multiple partners, substance abuse, trading sex, and not using condoms or other forms of contraception.

Based on information from Population Reports *(Heise, Ellsberg, and Gottemoeller 1999)*

However severe the physical consequences of violence, most women find the psychological consequences to be even more long-term and devastating (Sagot 2000). A recent World Health Report titled *Mental Health: New Understanding, New Hope* points to the disproportionate rates of depression among women and recognizes that GBV may contribute to these high rates (WHO 2001). Recurrent abuse can erode women's resilience and places them at risk of other psychological problems as well, such as post-traumatic stress disorder, suicide, and alcohol and drug use.

Health care providers can play a crucial role in detecting, referring, and caring for women living with violence. Abused women often seek health care, even when they do not disclose the violent event. While women tend to seek health services more than men throughout their lifespan, studies show that abused women seek services even more for ailments related to their abuse (García-Moreno 2002). Thus, interventions by health providers can potentially mitigate both the short- and long-term health effects of gender-based violence on women and their families. In Section II of this book, we will see the effects of these life-transforming and, at times, even life-saving interventions on the lives of women and their families affected by violence. ◠

Chapter Two

The "Critical Path" Studies:
From Research to Action

"It is said that we were all born under a star; when I watch the stars at night I ask which of them is mine, so that I can change it for another one."
—Quechuan woman, Peru

When PAHO's Women, Health, and Development Program developed its integrated strategy for addressing gender-based violence, it started out with an analysis of the problem. The "Critical Path that Women Follow to Solve Their Problem of Domestic Violence"[1] series of country studies and their results were instrumental in the strategy's development in many ways. The studies' action-oriented methodology provided vital information on women living in violent situations at the same time that it shed light on the types of local services (health, law enforcement, legal/juridical, educational, religious, nongovernmental, etc.) they most typically sought help from and in which sequence. It also revealed the most common obstacles they encountered from these institutions. Perhaps most importantly, the results of the studies served as a catalyst for raising awareness and mobilizing communities and policymakers to address the needs of women living in violent situations.

The need for such a study first arose from a series of women's health assessments that were carried out in the early 1990s by PAHO and its ministry of health partners in seven Central American countries.[2] The results identified GBV as a health priority within the study communities and highlighted the shortcomings and lack of coordination between existing services.

In response to this situation, PAHO and its multiple counterparts developed and applied the "Critical Path" qualitative research protocol. It was designed to catalyze the construction of an integrated strategy for addressing GBV that targeted women living in violent situations and incorporated local community resources and the social sectors–particularly the health sector–in a coordinated response to the problem. Its results provided community and national stakeholders with a much deeper understanding of the barriers that women faced in breaking their silence and in overcoming the obstacles, humiliation, and inadequate responses they encountered along their critical path.

The "Critical Path" results piloted 16 networks in 10 countries and stimulated national attention in each case. The health and other sectors responded by developing and implementing care procedures and protocols, training services providers, and setting up information systems to better detect and respond to GBV within the respective service centers. Moreover, in each country results were published and presented in national fora with policymakers, reinforcing the commitment to improve national policies and legislation that could address the alarming problem.

These first "Critical Path" studies entailed a lengthy research process that delayed the immediate use of the data by the communities. As a result, the protocol was simplified for its easier and more flexible application. The more streamlined "rapid assessment protocol" (RAP) has since been applied in many more communities, where its more readily available results inform their plans for addressing GBV issues (PAHO 2002). The Spanish and English versions of the original protocol and the RAP, the publications of country results, as well as of case studies of the 10 countries in Spanish,[3] are available through the PAHO Women, Health, and Development Program's Web site at www.paho.org/genderandhealth. The information provided in this chapter is largely based on the study results compiled in the 10 country case studies (Sagot 2000).

WHY THE "CRITICAL PATH"?

Information is key for identifying and addressing GBV, yet widespread under- and non-reporting continue to contribute to the problem's invisibility. The 2000 United Nation's report *World's Women* estimates that only 2% of sexual abuse among children and between 20% and 30% among women are reported (United Nations 2000). The "Critical Path" starts to bridge this gap by providing baseline information on the characteristics of women living with violence and the factors that motivate them to search for solutions. At the same time, it identifies the kind of responses by institutions that influence women to take or avoid taking the first steps on their path (Figure 2-1.).

---

1   "The Critical Path" research protocol was initially published in Spanish and then translated into English with the title Women's Way Out. For the sake of maintaining the concept of the critical path that women follow to escape their violent situations, the shorter title "Critical Path" will be used to refer to the research protocol and the study. Also, the term "gender-based violence" will be used instead of "family" or "domestic violence," unless the later forms part of a formal title or quoted definition.

2   The "Situation Analysis of Life Conditions with a Gender Perspective" (ASIS) and the "Diagnosis of Social Actors Working to Prevent Intrafamily Violence" were carried out in all seven Central American countries with support from the Governments of Norway and Sweden.

3   The original "Critical Path" protocol was developed by Monserrat Sagot and Elizabeth Shrader, who also coordinated the research process in the 10 countries. Sagot compared the results of the countries in La ruta crítica de las mujeres afectadas por la violencia intrafamiliar en América Latina: estudios de caso en diez países (2000).

FIGURE 2-1. **DIAGRAM OF THE "CRITICAL PATH"**

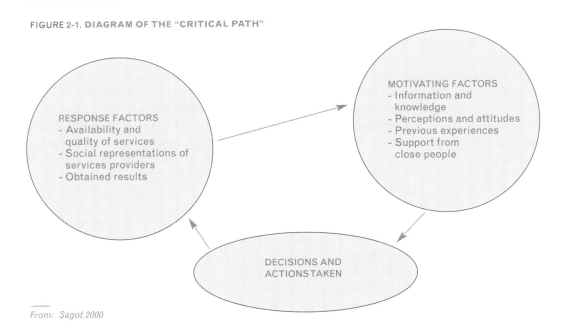

From: Sagot 2000

In addition to helping women and communities break the silence, the "Critical Path" also facilitates the coordination of responses that is essential for effectively addressing this complex problem. First, it helps women analyze and reconstruct their own experiences and empowers them to seek solutions within their own communities. At the same time, the research process helps community members and institutions to become more aware of their own shortcomings in responding to the needs of abused women, while motivating them to work together to achieve this common goal.

THE "CRITICAL PATH" METHODOLOGY

The "Critical Path" study was carried out in 16 communities of the 10 countries that were included in the two PAHO projects to address gender-based violence.[4] The study communities reflected the diversity of rural and urban settings in Latin America, as well

as that of its ethnic groups. Data were gathered between 1997 and 1999, and results were published in most countries by 2000.

The "Critical Path" uses an interactive, qualitative methodology with a standard protocol that was translated and adapted for the various ethnic groups. The process was guided by a set of pre-established ethical principles based on respect for the women's experiences as recounted, assurance of confidentiality and personal security, and a commitment by all participating institutions to the prevention and eradication of gender-based violence.

Information was collected through in-depth interviews with the women and semi-structured interviews with service providers in the health, law enforcement, legal/judicial, education, religious, and NGO sectors, as well as through focus groups with community

---

4   *The study was initially carried out in one community of each of the Central American countries and in three communities in each of the Andean countries as part of the PAHO gender violence projects. These will be reviewed in Chapter Three and were carried out in Central America with support from the Governments of Norway and Sweden, and in Bolivia, Ecuador, and Peru with support from the Government of the Netherlands.*

members. PAHO and its ministry of health counterparts selected the study communities based on size, the availability of basic services, and the existence of NGOs and/or women's organizations. From each community, participants included 15 to 27 women, aged 15 years or older, who were presently experiencing gender-based violence and who had contacted a service provider within the previous 24 months. A minimum of 17 providers from among the various types of service centers were interviewed in each community.

Data analysis was based on the interpretation of structured questionnaires. Interviews were recorded and transcribed for detailed analysis. The researchers worked closely with community teams to develop their skills and knowledge for collecting, analyzing, and utilizing the results.

FINDINGS OF THE "CRITICAL PATH" STUDIES IN THE 10 COUNTRIES

Even though the study included women from different countries and socioeconomic and ethnic groups, their experiences were tragically similar. Common characteristics included a general unawareness of their rights and the fact that most had taken at least some initial steps toward resolving their situation and had met with frustrating results. All experienced violence as a control measure being wielded by their intimate partners to reinforce the unequal power relationships within the family and the aggressor's own position of impunity.

"One of the issues is the machismo in our culture that says that a man is the strongest and has to be, in whatever manner, over a women, and when something does not suit him, he just beats her."
—Justice of the peace, El Salvador

In the comparison of the "Critical Path" studies of the 10 countries, Sagot provides a comprehensive and touching review regarding the common experiences of many different types of women (Sagot 2000). She quotes at-length from heart-wrenching accounts of women living lives enclosed in violence, and of their resourcefulness, courage, and strength in dealing with their situation, both within their families and when seeking help in their communities. Significantly, the majority of these women did not consider private or public services as part of their path, either because they were unaware of the support these institutions could provide, or because they had received inefficient or humiliating treatment by these groups in the past.

"The bureaucracy! Can you imagine? A person abused by her husband goes to the police station, then has to go to a forensic doctor, then back to the police, then to the district attorney's office; everything is such a mess. . . . "
—"Critical Path" report, Peru

"I report this case to the authorities, who then do nothing with him. They're not going to lock him up for the rest of his life. They're not going to heal my leg. . . . And if they would only lock him up for a day or two to teach him a lesson! I know they won't punish him."
—"Critical Path" report, Costa Rica

HIGHLIGHTS OF THE "CRITICAL PATH": THE WOMEN'S FIRST STEPS

All women interviewed identified GBV as a serious problem affecting their lives. They all reported being subjected on a regular basis to physical violence that included slaps, punches, and beatings, but some were also threatened with knives and guns, thereby placing their health and lives at great risk.

"He punched me again. He struck me on the temple, was on the verge of strangling me. It took me two months to recover, to be able to swallow again, and once again I ended up with a swollen and black eye."
—"Critical Path" report, Honduras

"He tried to kill me twice. The third time I think he will succeed."
—"Critical Path" report, Belize

Physical violence was almost always accompanied by psychological abuse. Yet, for however damaging and humiliating women described their physical and sexual abuse to be, they deemed the psychological violence to be even more painful, since it targeted their sexuality, self-worth, and parenting ability. Violence that included threats to their children was especially traumatic:

"He tells her: 'you are stupid [crying]), you are worthless and useless,' and she was only a year old. Then he tells me: 'look at your baby. She is worthless and stupid; you do not respect her.' . . . She was only a year old; she couldn't even talk yet; so she just stared at him, taking it all in."
—"Critical Path" report, Guatemala

"Because of the abuse my uterus was removed. . . . He continues to hit me, now always on the face, but what hurts most are the insults. I'm telling you, they are worse than if he had put a dagger in my back."
—"Critical Path" report, Peru

Most women also suffered sexual violence, but many were not aware of this abuse during most of their relationships, since they considered forced sex to be part of their domestic obligations.

"First he beats me, and afterwards he has sexual relations with me."
—"Critical Path" report, Guatemala

"When I was his girlfriend, he would tell me to go to his room. . . and I would be afraid. Then, one time, he pulled my panties down and got on top of me. I just thought this was the way things were. After that, whenever I would go there, he always did the same thing. It has always been like this. Talking with other people, I have been told that men caress you, but I don't know anything about that."
—"Critical Path" report, Guatemala

Intimate partners often subjected women to economic violence by limiting, withholding, or withdrawing financial support from them and their children, by threatening or actually by throwing them out of the house, by controlling any income the women brought home, and by breaking objects of value to the family.

Aggressors were men from all generations and all types of relationships, though the majority were intimate partners.

"The type of violence I see the most is that between husband and wife, because husbands don't really feel part of the marriage. They are good-timers, they are *machista*, they go out with women they find on the street, they don't take care of the home. When they do come home, there are problems. . . ."
—Health worker, "Critical Path" report, Panama

For a few women the abuse began immediately after establishing a relationship with their partners. For the majority, however, the violence started following cohabitation or marriage, a point at which their partners' behavior became markedly more aggressive. From that point these men were able to establish complete dominance over their partners and their sexuality.

"The problem started when we got married."
—"Critical Path" report, El Salvador

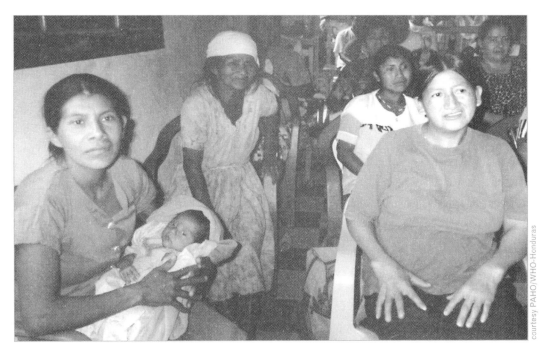

courtesy PAHO/WHO-Honduras

Honduran women attend a community meeting to learn more about GBV.

"Before he was different; he didn't so much as break a plate. But once he felt that he had his little chickie in his hand, he said: 'now the claws come out,' and he became a different person."
—"Critical Path" report, El Salvador

In many cases, the aggression had been long term, often starting or escalating during the first and subsequent pregnancies. Abuse during pregnancy not only resulted in abortions and sterility for the women, but also placed the lives of their unborn children at extreme risk.

"His intentions were to pull my baby out of my belly, because he put his knees on my belly and mistreated me."
—"Critical Path" report, Nicaragua

"I am eight months pregnant and when he comes home, he starts to rail and break up things. He kicked me in my belly, and the water bag burst."
—"Critical Path" report, Belize

Some women also reported having been abused by other members of their families, or by priests or teachers, even during childhood. Some young women reported entering into relationships, often with older men, to escape the abuse they experienced from their families.

"Well, if you can imagine, at the age of 8, to be exact, I was raped by my older brother."
—"Critical Path" report, Nicaragua

"I have been abused by my father and brothers many times. Once, when I was 10 years old, my dad hung me from a tree because I ate a piece of cheese."
—"Critical Path" report, Peru

In isolated rural areas, aggressors could more easily control their women's freedom. These women were least likely to interact with neighbors and to have access to social services, and were, therefore, at a higher risk of harm from violence.

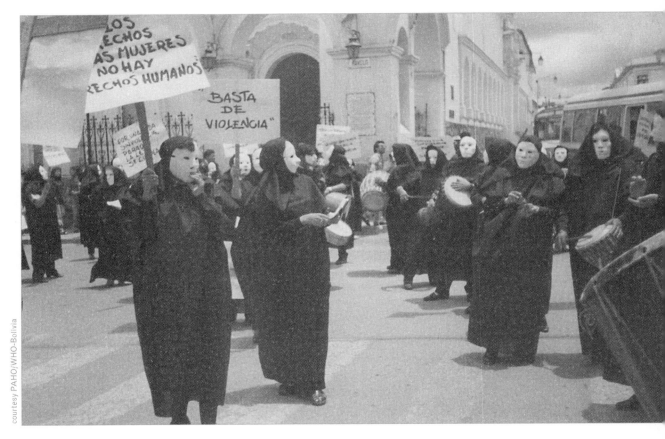

courtesy PAHO/WHO-Bolivia

Over the past decade, awareness by women of their civil rights has spread from large urban centers to smaller towns and villages around the Americas. This anti-violence demonstration by women indigenenous leaders in Sucre, Bolivia, has helped to promote violence prevention messages throughout the country and is spurring communities to view violence in a different way than in the past.

"For three years he kept me locked in a room. He opened the door at six in the morning to leave, and he wouldn't return until six in the evening. Not until that moment would I see the light of day."
—"Critical Path" report, Guatemala

Women often reported tolerating abuse because they feared that resistance might only intensify the situation. Staying in the relationship was also often encouraged by social pressures from their own mothers, children, and other community members in order to keep the family together. Lack of independent financial resources and family and institutional support also inhibited their actions.

"My face was bruised for a long time, perhaps a month. I didn't pursue the case because he told me that he could always get out of prison, but I would never get out of the cemetery. And I didn't want to die."
—"Critical Path" report, Honduras

"I've been patient because I feel sorry
for my children. To leave them or take them
with me would be worse, wandering about,
because I don't have a place to go with them.
That's why I've put up with so much from him."
—"Critical Path" report, El Salvador

"My parents told me: 'If he is your husband,
you just have to put up with the situation;
that is the way it is.' Then my mother said:
'This is how I have suffered with my husband, too.' "
—"Critical Path" report, Peru

The women tended to tolerate their violent
situations until they came to the realization
that their coping strategies were not
working and that their partners would not
change. They were especially motivated
to take the first steps when they perceived
changes in the pattern of abuse, such as
when the violence escalated; there was
infidelity; their aggressors squandered
their support, income, or possessions;
and especially when the aggression was
aimed at their children.

"He had a gun, and he threatened me with it . . .
all the time it was: 'I am going to kill you, you
common whore! I am going to kill you!' So when
he fired that gun, then I really became afraid. That
is how I finally got the courage to go to the police."
—"Critical Path" report, Bolivia

"I left because he hit my boy. He threw a big
piece of sugarcane at him. I got very angry
because he threw that stick at my boy as if
he were an animal, and he knocked him down."
—"Critical Path" report, El Salvador

Reliable support from family members and
friends and gaining access to information
about gender violence helped motivate
women to take the first steps towards resolving
their situations.

"When the neighbors saw how my husband beat
me up, they told me that it just wasn't worth it
for me to stay. They encouraged me to leave him."
—"Critical Path" report, Ecuador

"Thank God for those advertisements!
When I saw them, I said: 'I have to find out
more; I have to leave; I have to find out what
can be done about this."
—"Critical Path" report, Honduras

Once women reached the point of being
able to analyze their futile and dangerous
situations, and to acknowledge that they
were tired of living in fear for their safety
and that of their children, they accepted
that they could not tolerate any more abuse
and were ready to take action. For most
women, the way out–their critical path–was
painful and extended, often with relapses
back into the relationship, while a few were
successful in their initial attempt and were
able to follow a straightforward course out
of their situation.

". . . I felt like I had to fight to defend my right
to live in peace, to find calmness, and to raise
my children without violence, so that they could
grow up normally and have normal marriages."
—"Critical Path" report, Costa Rica

". . . I took the decision because I felt like
I was drowning."
—"Critical Path" report, Honduras

"Because I don't love him any more, I want to
leave him. . . . I got desperate because I used to
love him even though he hit me. But now I don't
feel anything for him, and I don't want to be with
him anymore."
—"Critical Path" report, Guatemala

While the majority of the women's paths
taken out were convoluted and at times
contradictory, analysis of the study data
showed that their decisions to start the path

and the directions they chose to take were constantly guided by careful consideration of the possible risks and outcomes.

**ARE SERVICE PROVIDERS
PART OF THE PROBLEM?**
When asked why they did not include public or private services in their "critical path," most women identified as primary obstacles the negative attitude of these providers and their inability or unwillingness to meet their urgent needs. These attitudes caused women to feel frustrated and uncertain; they feared that they would again be victimized and that there would be impunity for their aggressors.

"Often women do not show any [physical] evidence of abuse, so their claims are not believed and they are treated poorly. Many times they are blamed before anyone hears their side of the story. That's why most women don't go to the police. "
—Police officer, Peru

"Opening up discussions regarding violence only seems to weaken the women's position. They feel coerced to accept the impunity of their aggressors and to forgive and forget, and even to respect these men."
—"Critical Path" report, Ecuador

During their interviews, almost all providers of health, legal, and police services confirmed that women often feared that seeking their services would somehow worsen, instead of improve their situation. At the same time, this group acknowledged adhering to tradi-tional, patriarchal views that gender-based violence is a private matter, one that in most cases was warranted, and for which women were often to blame.

Generally speaking, the providers accepted that they did not understand all the com-plexities of GBV. Few professed to be fully conscious of the extreme danger that

women in their own communities faced daily in their abusive situations or about the dire conditions that eventually drove them to seek help. Furthermore, the providers were rarely aware of the risk involved in initiating and adhering to a "critical path" out of violence, while at the same time, they expressed frustration that women rarely followed the straightforward paths that providers were likely to prescribe.

According to the women, the generalized lack of understanding on the part of service providers resulted in such antagonistic behaviors as indifference, questioning, mocking, and attempts to instill guilt; in extreme cases, even sexual harassment and collusion with the aggressors were noted. When they did respond to the women, the providers would rarely follow up their cases or refer these clients to appropriate services. As a result, the women would often give up in frustration in dealing with the labyrinths of "proof" they were required to provide in order to initiate criminal or judicial proceedings. Especially in dealing with the police and judicial systems, women in all the countries studied noted an overwhelming feeling of futility in ever seeing their civil rights protected and receiving justice for the wrongs committed against them.

**STEPS ALONG THE "CRITICAL PATH":
HOW WELL DID THE SECTORS RESPOND?**
➤ **The health sector:** Women's reactions to the care they received from this sector were mixed. While almost all of the women interviewed said that they had visited their community health center on a number of occasions for various conditions —some of them related to their abuse—they concurred that health providers rarely asked them questions about violence or screened them for it.

"Women see these [health] institutions as places where they can heal their wounds or illnesses, but not as the right place to talk about their violent experiences."
—Monserrat Sagot, 2001

"The staff here do not ask and do not have the proper training for detection; nor do they consider it to be part of their job."
—Health provider, Honduras

During the time of this study, only a very few health providers had received any specialized training in dealing with women living in violent situations, and none had protocols or standards for care. Perhaps for this reason, the women perceived a generalized reluctance by health workers to deal directly or in a sustained fashion with their problem. Most health personnel elected instead to refer the women to the police or local court system, fearing perhaps that treating and following up on these cases would ensnare them in extended legal processes for which they had no time and wished to avoid at all cost.

"We verify a rape with a relative. We are not interested in who did it, or how or where it happened because that is none of our business . . . it's a legal problem."
—Doctor, Ecuador

Furthermore, the study showed, most providers had no further contact with these women and were thus unaware of any subsequent treatment or assistance they received elsewhere.

➤ **Law enforcement and legal/juridical systems**: The police and legal services were, in many instances, the first places women went, whether on their own or upon referral by health workers or other service providers. Police stations were present in almost all the communities studied. They

were also the least supportive, in terms of the providers' attitudes and willingness to help and the availability of gender-sensitive services and information. This, combined with the fact that the police and juridical officials generally were not aware of laws to protect the women—nor did they apply them—caused great frustration and humiliation among the women in all the countries studied. This overall deficiency was further exacerbated by the lack of coordination between the various sectors when women sought help, causing additional delays and/or interruptions in the "critical paths" women attempted to take out of their situations.

"When women come and ask to reprimand their husbands, we don't even keep a record of the complaint."
—Policeman, El Salvador

"All in all, it's a very painful experience. Many times the women go to the police in tears, and the police tell them not to be irresponsible and waste their time, as if they didn't have anything else to do. Then they tell them: 'So be it missus, tonight your man will be between your legs again.' In other words, besides not helping them, they disrespect them."
—Legal services provider, Nicaragua

"In the long run, the person just gets tired of going from one place to the next. A woman is raped, and first she goes to the police, where they tell her this is a family issue. They arrest the character and make him pay a fine because they don't want to send the case to the court. So next she goes to a lawyer; then to the district attorney's office and the judge, and many times she's told there's not enough information to prosecute . . . so eventually she says: 'Okay, fine' . . . and just gives up and leaves."
—"Critical Path" report, Bolivia

➻ **Education sector:** Because gender and family violence are issues normally falling outside the domain of educational policies and curricula, schoolteachers understandably feel ill-equipped to respond to the needs of affected students and their families. Therefore, most teachers maintained a cautionary attitude that wavered between awareness of the problem and avoidance of becoming involved in legal issues regarding minors.

"Some of the other teachers told me: 'don't interfere, don't let yourself get too close, because sometimes when you try to do a favor, it can really complicate your own life.'"
—Teacher, Peru

". . . It is not the responsibility of our staff to become too deeply involved in the family problems of our students."
—Teacher, Ecuador

Some teachers, however, said they had provided support to students despite the lack institutional guidelines, and they expressed a desire to see violence-related issues better addressed in their schools in the future.

"In the absence of specific policies regarding violence, teachers have relied upon their own instincts and used their best judgment."
—"Critical Path" reports, Peru

➻ **Community organizations:** These groups would appear to be in the best position to detect and address GBV, principally because they are made up of townspeople who are involved in all aspects of local life. The analysis showed, however, that most conventional community organizations, such as labor unions and cooperatives, held traditional beliefs and provided no support at all to women affected by violence. Even in local businesses where women held leadership roles, these managers usually lacked the information, skills, and policies to detect and respond to the problem. On occasion, women did seek

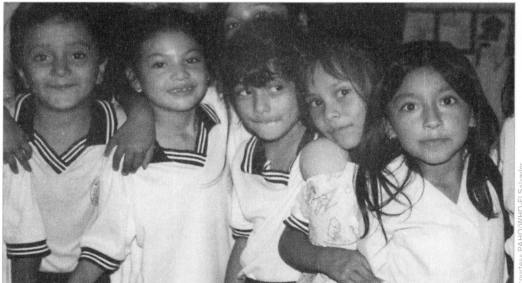

While still far from being the norm, some young schoolchildren, such as this group in El Salvador, have received information and discussed gender-based violence in the classroom with their teachers and other community members.

spiritual support to help them gauge their situation and justify their actions. Some religious organizations acknowledged an awareness that gender-based violence existed, but in their practices and counseling, they usually provided no specific support to affected women.

"A woman must count to three and swallow, so that the anger goes away and to avoid more aggressions."
—Priest, Ecuador

"I asked [the nun] if that was normal or what. . . . She told me that it was not normal, that it was a rape and that I did not have to say otherwise."
—Costa Rica

According to the interviews, women's organizations provided the best support, especially those which provided services related to women's health, legal rights, self-esteem, and other related issues. Groups of this type were often able to effectively meet women's needs, because their mission was to serve disadvantaged and abused women. Unfortunately, their support was limited mostly to larger urban areas and did not extend to rural communities.

". . . We listen to the woman and then put the ball back in her court: how would she like us to help her, we ask. . . . We treat those who seek our services with respect; we explain possible alternatives, but the decisions are theirs."
—Women's NGO, Honduras

LEARNING FROM THE "CRITICAL PATH"
In all 10 countries studied, the "Critical Path" results conclusively confirmed that GBV is a serious public health and human rights problem. They also indicated that as long as the problem remains largely invisible to and disregarded by society as

a whole, the social development of women, girls, their families, and communities everywhere will be compromised and diminished. The research process included a component in which the results were presented to the various sectors that had been interviewed. The women's stories, in particular, helped to "break the silence" regarding this complex problem and changed the attitudes of the study communities towards GBV by making their residents, and especially service providers, more aware of the tremendous burden placed on the numerous women affected due to the woeful inadequacies of services and national policies. This, in turn, spurred the communities to create concrete, intersectoral actions to address gender-based violence.

The analysis of the results of the "Critical Path" showed that the success of interventions depended on the availability, quality, and coordination of services, and, most of all, on the commitment of the providers. Women provided the most positive responses when they felt that the institutions, whether public or private, were genuinely concerned about their welfare, provided emotional support and information, respected and supported them, and showed a willingness to defend their rights and safety. They particularly appreciated the efforts of providers to help strengthen their self-determination and facilitate their ability to make their own decisions about when and how to free themselves from their violent situations. The services deemed most effective were those which remained unencumbered by rigid, institutionalized mandates and whose flexibility enabled individual situations and needs to be taken into account. To the extent to which the institutions exhibited these qualities, they were able to serve as valued stepping stones along the women's "critical paths." ⌒

Chapter Three

Joining Forces to Address Gender-Based Violence in the Americas

> ". . . Intimate partner abuse against women is a complex problem, from its causes to its consequences to its effective prevention. Only when we are convinced that our societies must be free from violence, can we embark on the path toward its abolition."
> —Cecilia Claramunt, 1999

In the early 1990s, as women's rights and the interrelationship between health and socioeconomic development gained new importance on international agendas, PAHO and its ministries of health counterparts in Central America carried out the first gender and health situation assessment, with support from the Governments of Norway and Sweden. The timing was especially relevant, since most countries were undergoing health sector reform processes to increase efficiency and decentralize services, without necessarily taking into consideration how these processes could affect men and women differently. Many women's organizations, therefore, feared that women might be further marginalized as a result of these reforms.

The assessment focused on the health situation of women, as well as the existing sources of care and information that could bridge the gender equity gap; it was carried out with health personnel and leaders in study communities in the seven Central American countries. Among the multiple inequities identified, the prevalence of and lack of response to gender-based violence emerged as the most urgent health need. The results also provided important clues as to the issue's complexity and suggested that an effective response could not be mounted by the health sector acting alone. These findings led to the "Critical Path" study reviewed in Chapter Two, which provided an in-depth view of the reality of countless women living with violence and of the institutions that could join forces to address the situation.

In response to these results and the 1993 PAHO resolution, PAHO presented its first proposal to address violence against women to the Nordic donors in 1994. The 1995–1997 project focused on women and girls in the 12–49 age group and on possible collaborations between the health sector and civil society. Soon afterwards, the Government of the Netherlands provided funds to implement this strategy in Bolivia, Ecuador, and Peru, as well.

The way the strategy was implemented varied according to the specific needs and situations of each locale, but all the countries addressed GBV at three levels—national policy, sector, and community—and in collaboration with partners. Allies were identified through a "Diagnosis of Social Actors Working to Prevent Intrafamily Violence" (1995) and through the research of the "Critical Path that Women Follow to Solve Their Problem of Domestic Violence" (1996).

The next phase of the Central America project (1998–2002) sought to consolidate this strategy and its prior achievements by institutionalizing the norms and protocols for the detection and care of victims, training community leaders and providers from the health and other sectors, and expanding networks and support groups for women and men to 30 communities. Due to internal policy changes, the Government of the Netherlands ceased its multilateral support for the Andean project when it ended in 2000, opting instead to continue with bilateral support for Bolivia (2001-2002) and Ecuador (2000-2002).

PUTTING THE PIECES TOGETHER

The "Lessons Learned" assessment and the yearly project evaluations credited the project's impressive achievements in large part to the strategy's targeting of outcomes from its conception and to the integrated partnership approach that had been applied at all three levels.

FIGURE 3-1. **THE INTEGRATED STRATEGY FOR ADDRESSING GENDER-BASED VIOLENCE**

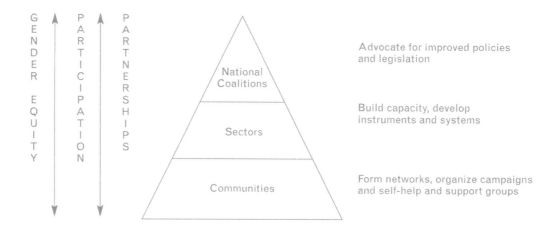

Figure 3-1. illustrates the three operational levels of this approach and the crosscutting values of gender equity, participation, and partnerships. The primary goal of this strategy is to put in place policies, capacities, systems, and networks to better detect and care for women who live with violence and to prevent gender-based violence by promoting a culture of peace, respect, and equity within families and communities. Each of this strategy's components has been carefully selected, based on research results, experience, and the process of negotiation. The values, interventions, and operational levels are briefly described below, and their applications will be more thoroughly discussed in the second half of this book.

CROSSCUTTING VALUES

→ **Gender equity:** Gender-based violence places women at risk of health problems and even death and is related to their inequitable socioeconomic status within their families and society in general. The resulting subordination and sense of powerlessness often thwarts women's ability to seek help and protection for themselves and their children. It is, therefore, important that policymakers, service providers, and community leaders be aware of these underlying inequities that affect women's human rights and health.

→ **Partnerships:** GBV is a complex problem that cannot be solved by the health sector alone. Its causes are multiple and interrelated, and therefore addressing them calls for a multisectoral approach. It is therefore imperative to create alliances at all levels with partners best suited to address these causes, such as the juridical, law enforcement, health, education, and social welfare sectors, as well as local political and community leaders and NGOs. Other key allies are the women's organizations that provide expertise,

accountability, and advocacy, and the national offices of women's affairs that formulate and monitor government policies.

→ **Active participation** by community stakeholders and beneficiaries provides the creative approaches and sense of ownership essential for formulating policies, developing networks, and changing the culture of violence.

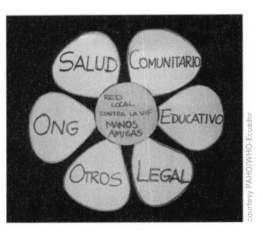

Training material prepared by Ecuadorian community network highlights the crosscutting values of partnerships and active participation that are key elements in the integrated approach promoted by PAHO.

INTERVENTIONS OF
THE INTEGRATED STRATEGY

→ **Detection** of abused women is the first step towards breaking the vicious circle of violence and preventing future and additional harm to the affected individuals. Since health providers are in regular contact with women, it is important that they learn how to screen for GBV on a regular basis (Chapter Six).

→ **Attention and care.** The solution to violence against women is neither straightforward nor exclusively medical. The number and variety of challenges women and their children face, presented in Chapters Five and Six of this book, make it imperative that providers be able to rely on effective policies, training materials, care protocols and procedures, efficient registration and referral systems, and the institutional support necessary to ensure the quality and specialized care that these clients need.

» **Promotion and prevention.** Raising awareness about gender-based violence, and the laws and services that address it, are key for preventing violence against women. Campaigns promoting gender equity, women's legal rights, and conflict resolution are the first steps toward creating a lasting culture of mutual acceptance and self-esteem for women and men. Incorporating gender issues, particularly those related to GBV, in school and university curricula raises collective awareness and helps prepare communities and professionals to more effectively address violence and its sequelae.

OPERATIONAL LEVELS OF THE INTEGRATED STRATEGY

» **Community level.** As described in Chapter Seven, the foundation of this strategy lies at the community level, where networks may be formed and encouraged to prevent, detect, and respond to violence against women. Health centers can play a catalytic role in mobilizing the community to develop these networks, in the sense that they can provide the training and set up the necessary surveillance and referral systems among the network's members. In many communities a simplified "Critical Path" survey has been conducted to identify stakeholders and the common obstacles women face when attempting to leave their violent situations. Network composition varies by community, but typically consists of the local health center, police station, court system, school-

teachers, community leaders, and women's organizations; in some communities church representatives and others participate, as well.

The networks usually develop work plans and meet regularly to coordinate activities. Bolivia (OPS 2000) and Peru (OPS 2001) have developed simple training manuals for use by networks, and members of the Central American project have also developed a strategic planning manual to guide this process (PAHO-Costa Rica 2001). Within their respective communities, networks organize and carry out campaigns against violence, provide information and support to families living with GBV, facilitate referrals, and coordinate training sessions.

"Now there is a lot more information on the radio and on TV; you know there are places to go, and if you get out before it's too late, they can save your life, and you can live in peace."
— *"Critical Path" report, Honduras*

As we will see in Chapter Seven, in an increasing number of communities, these networks have organized support groups for women and men that are commonly led by health center staff. Some members of these support groups have, in turn, taken the leadership to form other self-help groups within their communities.

» **Sector level.** In order to build capacity and set up the necessary systems to detect and care for abused women, public and

NGO sectors need to have access to specific policies and tools. In most of the project countries the health sector has taken a leadership role in making these available, while in some countries, this sector has coordinated with the local police department, women's NGOs, and/or universities for their development and implementation.

These sectors have worked together to publish modules and train health directors and providers—doctors, nurses, promoters, social workers, and others—as well as service providers from other sectors. The health sector has developed protocols and procedures for care that have been validated in the communities and provide an effective basis for training programs. As we will see in Chapter Five, currently the health sector is working with other sectors to refine registration and epidemiological data collection processes and thus facilitate better identification and tracking of cases of violence.

➤ **National policy level.** Stakeholders need to form cohesive alliances to advocate for policies and legislation aimed at preventing, treating, and penalizing violence, as well as for securing the resources for their implementation and continuous monitoring. In most countries, the health sector has allied with stakeholders from other sectors to form national and/or regional coalitions. These are described in Chapter Four.

During regular meetings, the coalitions share experiences; collaborate in developing policies, training materials, information systems, and other tools; and carry out national campaigns. They also assure that their respective achievements are sustained and institutionalized, which is

key for expanding the strategy to new areas throughout the country.

WHAT HAS THE PROJECT ACHIEVED?

By the end of the project's second phase (2002), the model strategy has resulted in the creation of more than 150 intersectoral community networks in 10 countries. In Central America, counterparts are using modules to train additional providers, have approved protocols and procedures, and are developing surveillance systems in all seven countries. These partnerships have strengthened national coalitions and enabled them to sustain advocacy efforts despite various changes of governments and health ministers. At the regional level, PAHO has joined forces with other United Nations agencies, regional women's organizations, and other partners to implement the international and regional conventions described in the introduction to Section I, and in 2001 it hosted a regionwide inter-agency symposium to identify priorities and formulate strategies for strengthening the health sector's response to GBV.

Constructing this integrated strategy has been the work of many groups and individuals. The process has been creative and innovative in the sense that it has brought together entities—the health sector, law enforcement agencies, the court system, educators—who in the past approached the issue of gender violence in different ways and did not always share the same perspectives and goals. The results, as shown in Table 3-1., could not have been achieved without the collective efforts of all these and other groups, working together at various levels and sharing a common commitment to break the silence surrounding an important public health and human rights issue. As a result, public interest and awareness have reached new heights. Now there is no turning back. ✎

TABLE 3-1. ACHIEVEMENTS IN ADDRESSING GENDER-BASED VIOLENCE IN 10 COUNTRIES, 1995-2002

1.REGIONAL LEVEL

- *Symposium 2001: Gender-Based Violence, Health, and Rights in the Americas*: 300 representatives of agencies, governments, and NGOs of 27 countries agree to a plan of action to mobilize the health sector to address GBV.
- *Technical exchanges* facilitated between Central American and Caribbean countries to expand GBV strategy to five Caribbean countries, as well as exchanges among 10 project countries on policy promotion, training of health personnel, and development of networks and support groups and of surveillance and information systems.
- *Political commitment:* GBV prevention placed on the agenda of regional and subregional policy fora and summits.

2.NATIONAL POLICY LEVEL

- *Advocacy:* Intersectoral coalitions formed in 10 countries to advocate for GBV policies and legislation.
- *Legislation:* GBV laws passed in 10 countries; monitoring bodies established in six Central American countries.
- *Research:* "Critical Path" results published in 10 countries; prevalence study on GBV and men's roles conducted in Bolivia; knowledge, attitudes, and practices study carried out in Peru.
- *GBV prevention campaigns* carried out in 10 countries.
- *Health sector reform:* GBV detection, care, and prevention policies incorporated in health sector reform processes of five countries.

- *Education:* Study of violence in primary school curricula in Belize and Peru, and in university-level curricula in Belize, Costa Rica, El Salvador, Nicaragua, Panama, and Peru.

3.SECTOR LEVEL

- *Strengthening capacity:* Instruments and systems developed and implemented (norms and protocols in 10 countries, surveillance systems in five countries, and training modules in 10 countries); more than 15,000 representatives from health and other sectors have received training each year of project period.

4.COMMUNITY LEVEL

- *Community networks:* Formation of more than 150 community networks comprised of health, education, and judicial sectors; police; churches; community leaders; and women's organizations.
- *Support groups* for men and women formed in five countries, community self-help groups in eight countries.
- *Zero tolerance campaigns* and other nonviolence activities promoted in numerous communities.

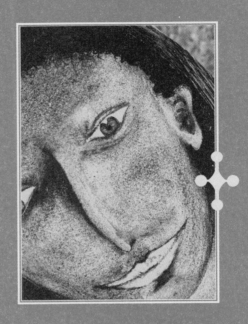

Women are waiting for
someone to knock on their
door; some of them have
been waiting for
many years. . . .
—Health provider, El Salvador

SECTION II
Lessons Learned from Central America

INTRODUCTION

In 2001, as the second period of Nordic funding for PAHO's Central American GBV project was coming to a close, there was consensus among PAHO, the donors, and national partners that the time had come to assess the actual achievements of the project before moving forward.

It was already obvious from yearly meetings with national project partners and project reports that a great deal had been accomplished in the last seven years: laws had been reformed; policies on violence had been implemented in many countries; countless providers had been sensitized to the issues of violence; registration forms for tracking violence had been developed; and community networks had been established. However, it was not possible to determine from these meetings and reports what difference these activities had actually made in the lives of women and their families who had been affected by violence.

The Norwegian and Swedish international cooperation agencies NORAD and Sida were particularly interested in carrying out an overall assessment of the project's achievements, as well as of its impact, efficiency, and sustainability. In addition, PAHO was anxious to use the opportunity to provide a more in-depth view of what the impact of the project had been to date, in order to strengthen, and if necessary, reorient, future cooperation.

Specifically, the partners were interested in finding out whether the policy reforms and training efforts had changed the way health providers thought about violence and addressed it in their practice. Were they more likely to ask women about violence, and if so, did they feel more confident in their ability to respond appropriately? Did the project affect the overall quality of health services in any way? Had coordination between institutions dealing with violence been strengthened? Had the "critical path" that women followed to overcome violence become any less burdensome? Most importantly, how did women feel about the new role that the project encouraged health providers to take on? Did it help them feel safer or more empowered to deal with the violence in their lives?

Therefore, an important aim of the review was to identify the important lessons and advice that providers, activists, and policymakers, as well as survivors, could offer to others embarking on similar projects.

The Program for Appropriate Technology in Health (PATH) was asked to carry out the review, and the U.S. Centers for Disease Control and Prevention (CDC) provided technical assistance. Because the International Planned Parenthood Federation, Western Hemisphere Region (IPPF&WHR), was also initiating an evaluation of its own GBV project in the Dominican Republic, Peru, and Venezuela, the review team collaborated with consultants and representatives of IPPF as well as PAHO in the development of the methodology. Both in-depth qualitative and participatory methods were used, including:

1. a review of project documents, as well as documents produced within the project countries

2. interviews with key informants in each country, including:
- PAHO consultants
- ministry of health staff
- representatives of women's groups and institutions that work together in the area of violence

3. focus group discussions with various stakeholders, including:

➔ members of national level commissions to prevent violence

➔ health providers from local health centers

➔ community leaders

➔ members of community violence prevention networks

➔ clients of health services (women who had received individual services for violence-related problems or who had participated in support groups for victims)

➔ members of an offenders' treatment program (Honduras).

The selection of key informants was made jointly by PAHO and representatives of the ministries of health, and the focus groups were set up by the local health centers and community networks. In total, more than 300 individuals were interviewed through the following activities:

➔ visits to five countries

➔ 31 focus group discussions

➔ visits to 10 community project sites.

During the group interviews the review team used the following participatory techniques to stimulate discussion (Chapters Six and Seven present a more complete description of the methods used):

➔ "The Road Traveled" (a chronogram of collective histories)

➔ "Who Helps Rosita?" (Venn diagrams for institutional analysis)

➔ achievements and barriers (free-listing and ranking)

➔ "Rosita's Story" (story completion for the analysis of quality of care).

As much as possible, the same techniques were used with the different groups, in order to permit comparisons between the views of clients, service providers, and members of community networks. In each of the sessions, one member of the review team facilitated the session while another took notes. The diagrams produced in the groups as well as the notes were transcribed afterwards for analysis.

The fieldwork for the study was carried out during July and August 2001. Given the limited time available for the study, the team decided to focus on achieving a greater depth of analysis in a few countries rather than visiting all of the countries, but obtaining a more superficial view. Therefore, field visits were performed only in El Salvador, Guatemala, Honduras, and Nicaragua. In order to learn about some of the experiences of Belize, Costa Rica, and Panama, a joint meeting with PAHO and its country representatives was held in Costa Rica. The preliminary results of the review were presented in a seminar in Panama for representatives from PAHO, the partner countries, and donors in October 2001. Comments from all the participants were incorporated into the final report (Ellsberg and Clavel Arcas 2001), available on PAHO and Sida's Web sites (www.paho.org and www.sida.se, respectively).

The second section of this book presents the highlights of the evaluation, with an emphasis on the lessons learned by the project participants. It also includes some examples of project achievements from Bolivia, Costa Rica, Ecuador, and Peru, even though these countries were not included in the initial study.

The main constraints of this report are the relatively limited amount of time and space available to provide an in-depth view of such a broad topic. With the exception of Nicaragua, the time spent by the review team in each country was relatively short, and in some cases it was not possible to interview all of the key people involved in the project. Therefore, a debriefing seminar was held in Panama with PAHO and national counterparts in order to ensure that the study's findings would be placed within their proper context and to address any issues of concern or perceived shortcomings of the study.

Because it would be impossible to do justice to the wealth of information collected during the research for this book, the review team has tried to synthesize the findings as much as possible in order to present a global vision of the project's principle accomplishments and barriers. Section II will therefore highlight those aspects of the project that are common to all countries, as well as issues that are unique to a single setting. Whenever relevant, international experiences are also referred to. The team has relied as much as possible on the actual voices of the participants and indicates areas where consensus and discrepancies were observed. At the same time, the evaluators have attempted to clearly indicate which statements are views of the interviewees and when they reflect the team's own opinions.

The review team would like to acknowledge all of the individuals who provided support throughout the completion of this lessons-learned review. These include the PAHO individuals listed in this book's acknowledgments section and those from the ministries of health, national NGOs, and the Governments of Norway and Sweden. Their steadfast commitment and support have enabled the PAHO project evaluation to come to fruition.

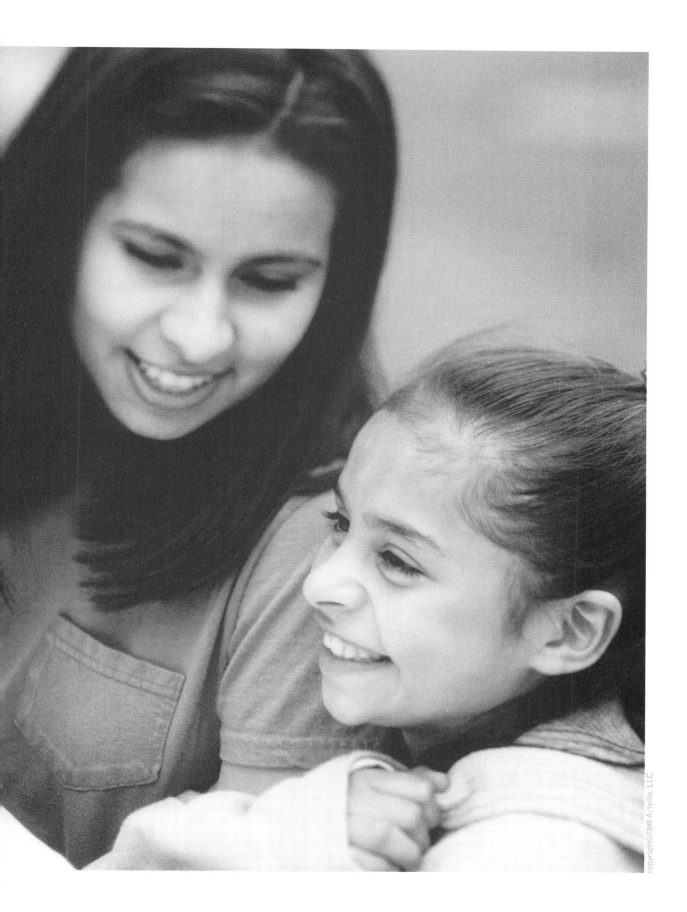

Chapter Four

Policy and Legal Reforms
on Gender-Based Violence

As pointed out at the beginning of this book, in the last decade there has been a dramatic surge in international recognition of violence against women as a human rights and public health problem. The Inter-American Convention on the Prevention, Punishment, and Eradication of Violence against Women, signed in Belem do Pará, Brazil, in 1994, marks a particular watershed for the Americas, as all countries in this Region committed themselves to making broad policy and legal reforms to address violence against women.

By the time of the PAHO project review in 2001, national committees had been established in all seven countries of Central America for the purpose of improving coordination and monitoring progress on the development of national plans and policies on violence. Most committees are headed by the national institutions for the promotion of women's rights and include representatives from the ministries of justice, education, and child welfare, as well as women's NGOs that work on violence. Initially, the health sector did not participate in these committees; however, now it has members in all countries with the exception of Guatemala. In Costa Rica, the health sector stands out as being the first state sector to establish a sector-wide plan for family violence; this step in 1994 served as the precursor for the subsequent development of PLANOVI (see Box 4-1.). The Ministries of Health in Belize and Panama have also played a prominent role in the development of national violence prevention programs.

One of the first goals of each of the committees was to achieve a basic agreement among the sectors to coordinate in a national violence prevention effort. In Costa Rica (PLANOVI 1994) and El Salvador national plans are already being implemented. In Belize, Guatemala, and Nicaragua national plans have been drafted but not put into effect. In Honduras and Panama, national violence prevention plans are currently being developed.

The creation of a national plan on violence against women is an important achievement in itself, as it creates a political space for greater dialogue between civil society and the state, at the same time that it commits governments to a public discourse that encourages sanctions against violence (see Box 4-2. on Peru's experience). Nevertheless, in most countries the transition from developing plans to putting them into practice

seems to be problematic. This is partly due to budgetary constraints, but at the same time these difficulties have political undertones. In Nicaragua, the National Commission on Violence against Women carried out a highly participatory planning process on violence against women that resulted in an ambitious and comprehensive proposal. However, shortly after its approval, the proposal languished for lack of resources to implement it. A member of the committee commented:

"The Inter-American Development Bank has offered to finance the plan, but due to the lack of pressure by the government, the funds have not been disbursed. If this were really a priority for the government there would be 10 ministers calling the IDB every day to ask what's happening with the loan."

In other countries where there is little tradition of coordination between civil society

---

BOX 4-1. THE NATIONAL PLAN FOR THE CARE AND PREVENTION OF INTRAFAMILY VIOLENCE (PLANOVI) OF COSTA RICA

In 1994 a number of public and nongovernmental organizations drafted a national plan to address intrafamily violence against women. The plan reflected the need for a national policy that embodied the spirit of the work that these groups had carried on for many years in addressing the issue of violence against women in Costa Rica. After much lobbying, especially on the part of women's organizations, this plan became PLANOVI. In 1998 an Executive Order established PLANOVI as the country's official system for responding to violence against women and children that was called for in the Domestic Violence Law of 1996. This system is coordinated by the National Institute of Women (INAMU) and is made up of government and nongovernment organizations, including the health sector, that provide services and support to women affected by gender-based violence.

The goals of PLANOVI are:
- to implement an integrated system for detecting intrafamily violence and extrafamily sexual abuse, preventing aggression, and providing care to affected persons so that they may recuperate and begin living healthier lives free of violence; and
- to promote actions to change sociocultural patterns that encourage and justify violent behaviors and to instill nonviolent lifestyles that are based on respect for individual differences.

PLANOVI is considered a model plan by neighboring Central American countries because of its intersectoral membership and its effectiveness in coordinating training, the development of materials, and lobbying under the leadership of INAMU.

PLANOVI Annual Plan 1997

BOX 4-2. THE EXPERIENCE OF PERU: THE NATIONAL TASK FORCE FOR THE COMPREHENSIVE CARE OF FAMILY VIOLENCE (*MESA NACIONAL*)

For the first time in Peru, national ministries, civil society, and international agencies have achieved a coordinated, sustainable approach to the issue of family and gender-based violence vis-à-vis the formation of the *Mesa Nacional Multisectorial para la Atención Integral de la Violencia Familiar* (National Task Force for the Comprehensive Care of Family Violence). Current members include the Ministries of Health, Education, Justice, Interior, and PROMUDEH (Program for Women and Human Development); and the Flora Tristán Center, a nongovernmental organization. Other participating (but nonvoting) agencies are the Pan American Health Organization (PAHO), the United Nations Population Fund (UNFPA), and the United Nations Children's Fund (UNICEF). Coordination of the *Mesa* rotates every six months, giving all sectors the opportunity to manage the coalition's agenda.

In 1999, as the result of the Critical Path process, the official members and Peru's Attorney General signed a national agreement that mobilized political will at all levels. The decree also facilitated a consensus-building process that resulted in the formation of networks at different levels and in the coordination of services that respond to the needs of Peruvian women living with violence.

The coordination of the members' contributions and expertise has resulted in greater quality and efficiency of the programs and policies that address gender-based violence.

Accordingly, the *Mesa* has coordinated training programs for health and other sector providers and has established a national database of information, research, and surveillance results.

The model of the *Mesa Nacional* has been replicated in 18 departments (states) and in many of their respective communities. During this process, the various sectors have been able to overcome many long-standing obstacles and work together to support and care for those affected by violence. The decentralized *Mesas* have raised their communities' awareness about the existence of violence and have provided incentives to overcome this problem. Their efforts have been strengthened by the regular sharing of lessons learned and best practices among communities and departments.

Beginning in 1997, a number of communities started self-help groups of women affected by violence. Through the coordinated efforts of their *Mesas*, member institutions facilitated the training of these groups' coordinators from Lima, Cuzco, and Piura, which resulted in the formation of more than 40 women's, men's, and mixed groups that involve approximately 500 participants per year, the majority of whom are women.

Throughout this process, PAHO has played a leadership role in consensus-building, the formation of *Mesa* working groups, and the creation of community self-help groups.

María Edith Baca, PAHO|WHO-Peru

and the state, and even among state institutions themselves, reconciling the priorities of different sectors is, in and of itself, a considerable challenge. A further obstacle is the oftentimes poor coordination between the national committees and local networks.

RECENT LEGISLATIVE REFORMS IN CENTRAL AMERICA

In the last 10 years, there has been an important movement to reform the laws concerning gender-based violence. This has largely been a result of the efforts of national as well as international women's organizations, such as the Latin American Committee for the Defense of Women's Rights (CLADEM). The critical legal analysis and lobbying efforts of women activists have been crucial in raising awareness of the weaknesses of current legislation and the need for reforms.

Another contributing factor has been the growth of women's commissions in the national legislative bodies who have contributed, often through bipartisan efforts, to reforms in critical areas. PAHO has been a principal agent in facilitating this process by targeting women parliamentarians, political leaders, cabinet advisors, and even wider political spaces such as RESSCAD (meetings of Ministers of Health of Central America and the Dominican Republic) in order to exchange experiences and define priority issues for joint action. Its presence in national reform processes within and outside the health sector is part of its wider advocacy role to defend the right of women to be free of violence.

Although the initiation of the reform process has had similar roots in the different countries, the actual content of the laws is largely determined by the specific political circumstances in each nation. The

capacity of social movements and even women's commissions to influence the final content of legal reforms is often limited. In some cases, new elements were added to laws making them more discriminatory to women, such as a reference to "virtuous women" in the definition of sexual crimes in Panama's Domestic Violence Law, or the addition of a clause criminalizing the "promotion" of homosexuality in the Nicaraguan Reform of the Penal Code on Sex Crimes. Although the content of the domestic violence laws varies by country, there are some common features. The most important achievements of the legal reforms have been the following:

→ **the establishment of protective measures** (Belize, Costa Rica, El Salvador, Guatemala, and Nicaragua);

→ **expanding the concept of injury,** so that severe psychological damage, such as major depression or post-traumatic stress disorder resulting from abuse, may be considered a criminal offense (Nicaragua);

→ **establishing family ties as an aggravating circumstance** in the case of injury, which warrants the use of more severe, rather than weaker, penalties (Nicaragua); and

→ **changing the status of sex crimes and spousal violence to public offenses,** and broadening the definitions, as well as the sanctions, for rape and incest (Belize, Costa Rica, Honduras, Nicaragua, and Panama).

GAPS AND PROBLEMS IN THE NEW LEGISLATION

In most countries, even where reforms have been passed, there are still important gaps. For example, although the Panamanian legislation contains a number of important and innovative measures regarding violence prevention, the treatment of victims of abuse, and sanctions to offenders, it is still generally very weak in terms of offering protection for abused women and children. In other countries, the legal reforms have been primarily geared towards protection and prevention, as in Costa Rica, and few changes have been made in the area of sanctions. Belize and Nicaragua have possibly the most progressive and complete legislation overall, in terms of addressing issues related to prevention, protection, and sanction. Following are some examples of gaps and contradictions in terms of legal protection and sanctions for offenders that are still present in many Central American countries:

➔ **Many legislative reforms do not address sex crimes (rape and incest), which are still considered private offenses.** In Guatemala, for example, this means that only the victim can file charges against an offender. Many women, and particularly children, are reluctant to file charges, and given the lack of protective measures, it may be quite dangerous for them to do so. Moreover, in many countries rape in marriage is not recognized as a crime. In the case of incest and spousal abuse, fear or family pressure often prevent women from reporting these crimes, or once reported, the charges are often subsequently dropped. This is considered by Guatemalan women's rights activists to be a serious constraint:

". . . We want sexual offenses to be officially prosecuted and incest to receive real sanctions. In Guatemala, incest carries a fine of 300-600 quetzales [US$ 40-90], and the aggressor can go free right away. . . . "
—Member of the Guatemalan Violence Prevention Commission, CONAPREVI

➔ **Witnesses are often required to corroborate the crime,** which in the case of spousal abuse and rape is rarely possible.

➔ **Penalties for injuries and sex crimes are often very low,** and quite often can be exchanged for a court pardon or for minimal fines.

➔ **In some countries, such as Honduras, arrests can be made only after a criminal investigation has been concluded,** which means that the woman who reports spousal abuse must wait up to two days before the police can make an arrest, during which time the abusive husband may still be living in the house with her.

➔ **Legislation which restricts women's access to family property or which does not guarantee men's obligation to provide child support keeps women in abusive relationships for reasons of economic dependency.** An example of progressive legislation in this respect is that of Honduras, where in the case of separation of common property, the house may belong to the husband, but everything inside it by law belongs to the wife.

PUTTING THE LAWS INTO EFFECT

Legislative reform is only the first step in developing effective strategies against gender-based violence. It is equally important to ensure that the justice system applies the laws correctly, and that women and children have a sufficiently adequate understanding of the legal system to be able to demand that their rights be safeguarded.

This is a weak area in all of the countries studied, where in many cases judges and police have little or incomplete knowledge of laws, and for various reasons do not apply them appropriately. In many countries the specific criminal procedures to be followed in applying the new laws are not yet clear. Furthermore, there appear to be many difficulties in establishing effective coordination between the law enforcement

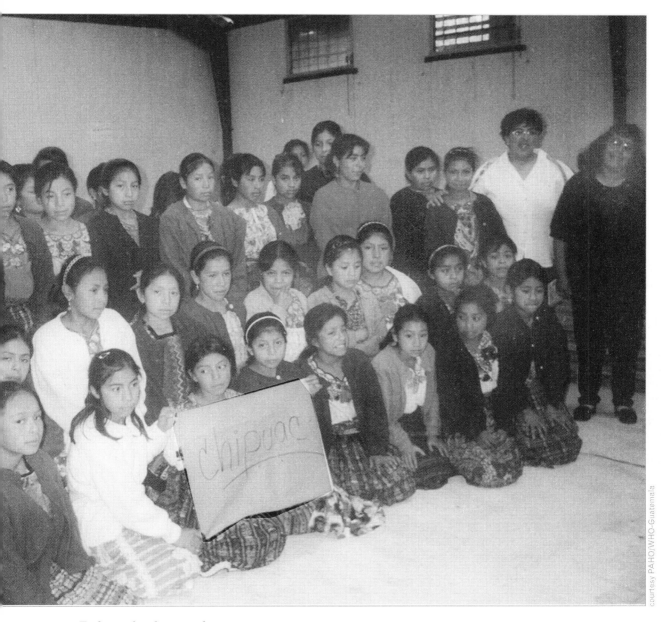

Teachers and students attend
public forum on violence
prevention in Guatemala.

and judicial sectors, both at the local and national levels. Following are examples of some of the weaknesses found:

➻ **Interpretations of the law are often based on cultural norms that are tolerant of violence against women and children.** For example, in Costa Rica, being under the influence of "a violent emotional state" is considered to be an extenuating circumstance for the crimes of homicide and injury, and legal experience in gender-based violence has shown that many judges interpret "jealousy," "heated discussions," anger, and infidelity as legitimate causes for such a state.

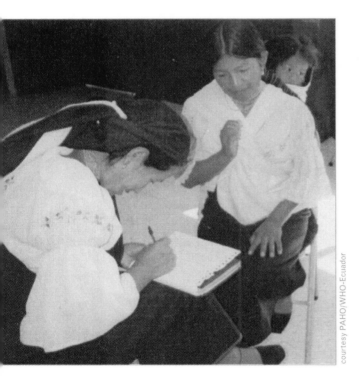

Women receive information about their basic civil rights in Ecuador.

This means that even when new laws are passed sanctioning GBV, it is much harder to change the logic under which the laws are applied. In Nicaragua, Justices of the Supreme Court have displayed biases in favor of offenders with such public statements as "If a man hits a woman, she must have done something to deserve it," and "A man who beats his wife must have a good reason for it; surely she did something to provoke it" (Ellsberg, Liljestrand, and Winkvist 1997).

This belief is not exclusive to judges, but rather permeates the attitudes and practices of other public officials, such as police officials, human rights ombudsmen, and public prosecutors in charge of investigating and processing charges of violence. This mindset often affects judgments on the criminality of a given act, especially when the only evidence is the victim's testimony. This is especially critical in the case of sexual abuse of children, where the main evidence is usually testimonial in nature.

➻ **There is little coordination between family courts and criminal justice courts.** Where they exist, family courts are usually in charge of issuing protective orders, whereas criminal courts are mandated to handle criminal proceedings against offenders. This means that, in practice, women are required to follow separate procedures for what, nonetheless, constitutes a criminal act, which in turn often produces contradictory and inequitable results. At the same time, women typically receive very little guidance to help them comprehend and successfully navigate the bureaucratic processes required for their complaint to be addressed.

➤ **There is a risk of contradiction in the application of family law and domestic violence legislation.** Many Central American countries have recently passed family codes, which generally establish the preservation of the family as a primary goal. The spirit of this legislation can be contradictory to that of domestic violence legislation, which has the goal of protecting the physical and moral integrity of individuals within the family. In practice, what this means is that whenever judges rule according to the principal of family unity, women will be obliged to remain with their abusive husbands, particularly in countries where effective protective measures are not in place.

➤ **In Honduras and Panama, the new laws establish the possibility of allowing offenders to receive "curative treatment" in lieu of prison sentences.** There is a great deal of controversy regarding the effectiveness of short-term psychological treatment in "curing" violent behavior (this issue will be addressed more thoroughly in Chapter Seven). However, a further constraint is that neither the Honduran nor the Panamanian public health system currently has established norms for the treatment of offenders, nor the capacity to carry out large-scale treatment programs.

➤ **Mediation is neither forgiveness nor reconciliation.** Another common problem is the use of mediation or out-of-court arrangements (*fianzas de paz* or *arreglos extrajudiciales*) for domestic and sexual violence situations. Mediation has become popular in many countries as a means to expedite solutions for misdemeanor offenses. However, when used in domestic violence or rape cases, it can be counterproductive because there are few guiding rules or principles for performing media-

tion, and therefore the agreements are subject to the individual interpretation of each police officer or judge. In Guatemala, as the indigenous women activists of Cobán explained,

"...The deputy mayors in the indigenous communities often use mediation as a way to make couples reconcile, because the focus is on sustaining the family at all cost. . . . "
—Cobán promoter

Although in Nicaragua, mediation is not officially allowed to be used in cases of violence and sexual offenses, several judges acknowledged that it frequently is applied. One difficulty with mediation is that it assumes that both parties are negotiating under equal conditions; however, this is clearly not the case when a woman has been beaten or raped by her intimate partner. As a consequence, the agreements that result from mediation often disguise the aggression. They are usually registered as "marital disputes" rather than "assaults," and in return for a husband promising not to hit his wife, she is often asked to promise not to provoke her husband and maintain order in the household. The faulty premise behind this solution is clear: it implies that both parties are equally responsible; the husband for using violence and the wife for provoking him. As one Nicaraguan lawyer commented,

"It was such a struggle to get the police to stop using out-of-court agreements. . . . Now with judicial mediation the whole package has been transferred over to the courts, but the problem is the same."

In some countries, judges refuse to apply protection measures such as restraining orders for the aggressor, alleging that it violates his rights.

"...If I apply the protection measures of Law 230 [i.e., forcing the offender to leave the home], I am violating the aggressor's right to own property. . . . "
—Judge, Nicaragua

➤ **Mandatory reporting discourages health providers from asking questions related to violence, for fear of getting involved in court cases.** The laws in Costa Rica, El Salvador, Guatemala, and Panama establish the obligation of public employees to notify the justice system if they become aware of cases of family violence. As a result, health personnel are reluctant to ask clients about violence and to register identified cases for fear of becoming involved in criminal cases.

➤ **In many cases, legal proof of abuse is required by specially trained forensic physicians, of which there are very few in Central America.** PAHO advocates that the laws be modified to allow any trained doctor to perform this examination. Bolivia recently passed a law permitting this, and the Organization is working with the Universidad Mayor de San Andrés, the national university, in the development of a training manual for medical students in legal medicine.

The problems mentioned above have many serious consequences, but the most important of these is that:

➤ **women may be more reluctant to report violence,** either because they believe that nothing can be done, or because of fear of reprisals;

➤ **women and children may be exposed to greater risks** by reporting acts of violence when there are not effective measures to protect them; and

➤ **the impunity resulting from the lack of institutional response** reinforces the belief among abusive men that they are allowed to beat their intimate partners and children.

As we have seen in this chapter, the increased international and regional attention that has been focused on gender-based violence as a social justice issue and human rights violation, combined with the advocacy and commitment of principally women's groups to this topic, have raised public and political awareness of the need for national policy and legal reforms to protect women and children from violence and to provide them with legal instruments to redress wrongs committed against them, whether by their intimate partners or through incest or rape. However, the changes that will be required are not always clear, since they often conflict with issues of privacy, socialization practices, and long-ingrained cultural patterns. At the heart of this change will be innovative actions at the community level—the construction of viable intersectoral networks and sustained cooperation—supported by national political commitment to remove as many barriers as possible to the development of a new culture of mutual respect among men and women. The examples of Costa Rica, Peru, and Ecuador (Boxes 4-1., 4-2., and 4-3.) illustrate the various aspects and possibilities of this approach.

In the next two chapters, we will see how the health sector, through its human face—the actual health workers—can play a key role in caring for women affected by violence and in increasing the visibility of GBV through better awareness, training, and reporting of cases. ➤

BOX 4-3. THE EXPERIENCE OF ECUADOR: THE *COMISARÍAS ITINERANTES*

In Ecuador gender-based violence is officially recognized as a public health and a social justice problem, and the right to a life free from violence is established in the nation's Constitution. The *comisarías itinerantes*, or mobile support units, offer an innovative response to women affected by violence in rural and/or remote areas where access to health education and legal services is limited and/or inadequate. The principal function of these *comisarias* "on loan" from other jurisdictions is to increase awareness about Law #103, (titled Violence against Women and Families, approved by the Government in 1995), reduce the risk of gender-based violence, and protect affected community members by enabling women to receive social, psychological, and legal advice. Furthermore, the coordination between local officials and visiting *comisarías*, while lacking formal legal authority, facilitates the training and conscience-raising of local authorities, service providers, and the community. The *comisarías'* activities are carried out within health and legal service centers and include:

- carrying out campaigns and informing affected women, providers, and the community about all national laws and legal instruments, especially Law #103, and increasing access by the affected women to legal services;
- disseminating information and options for those women and families affected by violence;

- increasing access by the affected women to health care and improving the quality and sensitivity of health services that respond to intrafamily and gender violence problems;
- introducing intrafamily and gender violence issues into basic educational curricula at the community level; and
- facilitating the dissemination of emergency contraception as an alternative to unwanted pregnancies resulting from sexual violence.

This initiative applies the constitutional rights guaranteed to all Ecuadorians, especially women, to have access to:
- information on their human rights, and, in particular, about their sexual and reproductive rights, and to a life free of violence, as stated in Law #103;
- quality health services which address intrafamily and gender violence;
- *comisarias* in all communities; and
- participation in community activities related to the prevention and control of violence.

As a result of this strategy, the *comisaría* have contributed to greater visibility of gender violence in communities throughout Ecuador. Health services have stimulated the replication of this strategy, with increasing focus on the importance of strengthening mobile legal and psychological services as well.

Zaida Crespo, PAHO/WHO-Ecuador

Chapter Five

The Health Sector:
Building an Integrated Approach

This chapter highlights the most significant experiences and lessons learned from PAHO and its Central American partners after nearly a decade of work in developing an integrated public health approach for addressing gender-based violence. This approach, as discussed in Chapter Three, includes interventions at the macro level (policy and legislation), the health sector (both policy and services), as well as at the community level.

WHY IS GENDER-BASED VIOLENCE INVISIBLE IN THE HEALTH SECTOR?

International research has consistently shown that women living with violence suffer a wide range of serious physical and mental health problems and visit health services more frequently than non-abused women. Despite this, medical records rarely identify violence as a reason for medical consultations, and, as the "Critical Path" study confirmed, most health care providers do not consider violence to be an important issue in their work (Heise, Ellsberg, and Gottemoeller 1999).

Many studies indicate that women living in violent situations rarely reveal their situation spontaneously to medical personnel, even when seeking help for violence-related problems, such as physical injuries. Providers, on the other hand, rarely ask women whether they have suffered violence, even when there are obvious signs of abuse. The situation described by a Nicaraguan doctor in the "Critical Path" study is representative of most health services in Central America:

"There's simply no time to talk or perform special exams for women reporting violence. The quality of care given to a victim of violence is not even close to that given to a woman with other chronic conditions."

As in the "Critical Path" studies, women interviewed by the review team offered similar explanations for their reluctance to talk about abuse: they feel ashamed of the violence and that health personnel will not be interested in or concerned about their problems.

"I thought that there were just a few people living like this and that it was something shameful. . . . I thought it would be embarrassing for someone to find out that a man was hurting me this way."
—Ellsberg et al. 2000

Another barrier for disclosure is the fear of reprisals and economic hardship:

"Women do not speak for fear that [the husband] will be put in jail and then no money will come into the household. Also because they are afraid of him. They think, 'if I talk he will kill me, he will choke me. . . .'"
—Woman activist from San Cristóbal, Guatemala

In Guatemala, indigenous women expressed their mistrust of the health system in general, due to experiences of discrimination in their dealings with health personnel:

"People think that our [indigenous] costumes make us stupid. . . . [In the health center] we have to wait longer. They call the *ladinas* first and tell us to please step aside. We do it because of the language and our fear of not being able to express ourselves well in front of the health personnel. The *ladinas* nurses are not interested in us. . . . "
—Woman activist from San Cristóbal, Guatemala

Providers also described many barriers that kept them from asking their clients about violence. Some felt that women would be offended by the question or that they would not know how to respond or that the providers would not have the time or resources to treat her if she revealed that she had been abused. A Salvadoran doctor described his early experiences in screening for violence this way:

"Sometimes I ask a woman about violence, and right there she begins to cry; she becomes a sea of tears. She closes up, and I have to wait. When someone isn't sensitized he can get annoyed and think, 'Why did I even ask?' and, 'Now how am I going to get rid of her?'"

Providers worry that screening for abuse will add yet another burden to their already overstretched capacity. In the majority of health centers, caring for women suffering violence is not yet part of the professional profile, and there are no information systems in place that would allow them to justify the time spent on violence cases.

Providers' attitudes about violence are also shaped by prevailing cultural norms. A study carried out among reproductive health providers by the International Federation of Planned Parenthood in three Latin American affiliates found that many of these providers expressed attitudes that place blame for violence on women rather than on their aggressors. Over half felt that some women's inappropriate behavior provokes their partner's aggression. Nearly one-fourth felt that women do not leave violent situations because on some level they like to be treated with violence (Guedes et al. 2002).

During the project evaluation interviews, many health providers noted having experienced violence themselves. In most of the group discussions with these personnel, at least one disclosed having been beaten by a partner. A Nicaraguan nurse who had been abused described her experience this way:

"I wanted to get things off my chest but I felt rejected by the other health workers . . . they thought less of me and made me feel guilty. . . . I would have liked for them to have explained that there are laws and support centers for women; to make me feel safe, to tell me that I wasn't alone. . . . I wish they had said to me, 'How do you feel? This is not your fault. . . . I care about what happens to you. . . .'"

Although in the discussion groups participants did not mention having been violent toward a partner, a study conducted by PAHO and Nicaragua's Ministry of Health found that, in individual interviews with health professionals, several male doctors acknowledged having been violent with their partners, and several women disclosed having been victims of violence. This study, performed by the Nicaraguan Association of Men against Violence, noted:

"Health workers—doctors, nurses, health inspectors—are men first before they are health workers. As a result, they cannot escape from the *machista* socialization that all men receive from their environment."
—Ministry of Health, Nicaragua, 2001

Transforming the culture of silence and complicity around gender-based violence is consequently the overriding challenge for any effort to influence health policy and programs.

PAHO'S INTEGRATED APPROACH TO ADDRESSING VIOLENCE FROM A PUBLIC HEALTH PERSPECTIVE

Given the lack of relevant international experiences to guide the integration of GBV into health policy and programs, PAHO and its partner organizations have developed an integrated approach in Central America, as was described in Chapter Three. Using the findings of the "Critical Path" research as a point of departure, this approach is being adapted and implemented in each country, integrated into the work of local stakeholders, and grounded in a thorough assessment of national and local realities.

In this sense, instead of promoting a "one-size-fits-all" model for addressing gender and family violence, the hallmarks of PAHO's approach have been flexibility and respect for local experiences. The project has sought to strengthen ongoing processes in each country, while encouraging the adoption of a basic set of guiding principles through technical collaboration, international meetings, and exchanges between countries. For example, the Honduran violence prevention model is based on the establishment of 13

Family Counseling Centers (*Consejerías de la Familia*), or FCC, located in regional health centers throughout the country. Each FCC has at least one social worker and psychologist and provides individual and group counseling for victims of violence, as well as training and prevention activities for health workers and community promoters. The Mental Health Department of the Honduran Ministry of Health manages the FCCs. In contrast, the cornerstone of Nicaragua's violence prevention model is the Women and Children's Police Stations (*Comisarías de la Mujer y la Niñez*), led by the National Police Force. In every city where a *Comisaría* exists, the local health services participate in a broad-based support network of governmental and nongovernmental organizations.

Despite national differences, the PAHO project has supported a series of common activities in each country, as well as international conferences and exchanges between countries, in order to encourage coherence at a subregional level. These include:

→ the development of national policies recognizing violence as a public health problem and outlining basic principles for caring for victims of violence from a human rights and gender framework (see example of Costa Rica's approach in Boxes 5-1. and 5-2.);

→ the drafting of norms and protocols that define the kind of care that should be offered, by whom and how; as well as defining mechanisms for monitoring activities;

→ the development of a training plan for personnel on the use of the norms;

→ the creation of support groups for violence survivors;

→ the promotion of male involvement in violence prevention activities;

→ the development of an information system that permits tracking reports of GBV throughout the health system;

→ the development of community-level public awareness to promote nonviolent lifestyles; and

Clinics that offer care for women living with abuse, such as this one in Ecuador, can play a pivotal role in reinforcing their clients' self-esteem and courage to continue on their "critical path" by simply providing a secure setting where the women may be heard, receive assurance they are not alone and are not to blame, and be provided with advice on how best to protect themselves.

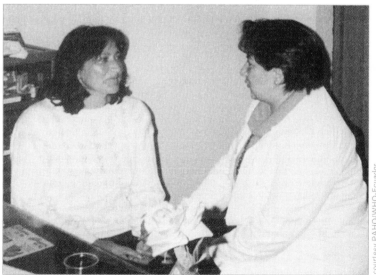

courtesy PAHO/WHO-Ecuador

➡ the establishment and/or strengthening of community networks to coordinate services and violence prevention activities.

In each project country at least one community was initially selected for piloting the integrated approach. During the second stage of the project over 150 communities throughout the subregion implemented the approach. In some countries it has been possible to leverage other national and international resources in order to scale up the project to include even more geographical areas. The following sections describe some of the main achievements and challenges encountered by the project assessment team with regard to GBV policies and norms.

HEALTH SECTOR GBV POLICIES: HOW IMPORTANT ARE THEY?
One of the early aims of the PAHO project was to encourage the ministries of health in partner countries to adopt explicit policies addressing GBV. To date, all of the countries now have some kind of national policy statement regarding family violence and/or violence against women. In some cases the policies were achieved through specific

Ministerial Decrees (Nicaragua), and in other countries the legislative reforms on family and sexual violence stipulate the role of the health sector in violence prevention. In El Salvador, there was no specific health policy related to gender-based violence at the time of the review; instead, it was included in the specific policy guiding the integrated care for families. In Guatemala, family violence is a subprogram nested within the Mental Health Program.

The policies are usually fairly general and simply state that:

➡ sexual and physical violence against women and children is a serious public health problem;

➡ health services should provide basic care for victims of violence; and

➡ providers should coordinate with other state institutions and nongovernmental organizations to ensure an integrated approach for the care of victims and in violence prevention activities.

The national policies on violence are potentially strategic tools for stimulating greater sensitivity among health providers and program managers about the issue and for forging a collective awareness among personnel that violence is an important public health issue that all providers need to address. However, in many countries where GBV health policies exist, they have not been widely disseminated, and there is still a large contingent of health workers who do not know about them.

WHAT IS THE MOST STRATEGIC PLACEMENT FOR GBV PROGRAMS WITHIN THE HEALTH SECTOR?
The experience of Central American programs indicates that where the program is

> ### LESSONS LEARNED
> The establishment of a specific health sector policy outlining the role of health providers in addressing violence is a key step towards institutionalizing violence programs and raising awareness among personnel.
>
> However, it is not enough to develop appropriate health sector policies on violence: it is equally important to disseminate them as widely as possible among health workers, as well as the population at large, so that the health sector can be held accountable for policy implementation.

placed within the health sector can have a profound impact on program implementation. From a policy perspective it is strategic to have the GBV program placed at a sufficiently high level organizationally so that it may influence overall planning and health sector reforms. In Costa Rica, and initially in Nicaragua, the GBV programs have been managed from the Planning Division of the Ministry of Health. This placement may be strategic for raising the profile of GBV at the national level and promoting inter-programmatic coordination. However, because the planning departments are generally not closely linked to hospital and primary care services, it may be more difficult to integrate GBV services into programs that are based in other ministerial divisions, such as those for mental health and reproductive health programs.

In most of the project countries, GBV and family violence programs are located either in the national departments for women's, maternal child, or reproductive health (Belize, El Salvador, Nicaragua, and Panama) or in the mental health programs (Guatemala and Honduras). Because gender-based violence affects many different aspects of women's lives, ideally, interventions to prevent violence and mitigate harm should be as broad as possible in their scope. For example, PAHO's experience indicates that including GBV programs in national reproductive health programs can facilitate the integration of GBV services into core reproductive health services such as prenatal care and family planning, as well as enabling their expansion throughout the primary health network.

The experience of Guatemala, on the other hand, exemplifies the challenges of addressing GBV when it is placed organizationally within mental health services. At one time the family violence program in Guatemala was situated in the maternal and child health division of the Ministry of Health. Due to ministerial reorgan-

> ## LESSONS LEARNED
> The placement of program coordination for care for gender-based or family violence in the areas of women's health and reproductive health services facilitates lateral integration into other programs and services.

ization the program was discontinued and has only recently been resurrected within the mental health division. Despite efforts by the mental health division to rebuild the program, some authorities acknowledge that the change has weakened the program. "Mental health is a virtual program," commented the director of a large health district in Guatemala that does not have a single psychologist. In Honduras, as well, where dealing with GBV is the exclusive domain of the Family Counseling Centers, its integration into maternal and child health and other health programs has faced similar challenges due to restraints imposed by organizational structure.

In contrast, reproductive health services, such as family planning and prenatal care, are available throughout the health system, even in the smallest health posts. There is generally technical support and supervision for the program at the district level, as well. Therefore, by integrating GBV laterally into reproductive health programs, it is possible to extend the scope of the program widely with relatively little additional investment.

Moreover, because reproductive health services are available in virtually every health care setting everywhere, no matter how modest or sophisticated, integrating care for GBV in these basic services increases the quality of care in the programs, as well. In contrast, mental health services are generally scarce, are usually found only at the regional level or at specialized referral clinics, and are therefore able to reach only a small proportion of women living with violence.

BOX 5-1. PRINCIPLES TO GUIDE CARE FOR SURVIVORS OF FAMILY VIOLENCE

- Family violence is a serious problem that affects the physical, emotional, and sexual health of the person that lives with it and her/his family and can even lead to death.
- Family violence is a criminal offense with legal repercussions; therefore, it should be addressed in a timely and effective manner.
- Family violence is the responsibility of all society, as well as a public health and human rights problem.
- Violence is caused by the perpetrator, not the victim.
- Violence is a learned behavior, and, therefore, it can be unlearned.
- Nothing justifies family violence.

- People have the right to live under conditions that allow their integrated development and respect for their rights.
- All individuals, regardless of sex, age, religion, economic level, sexual orientation, nationality, and political beliefs, should be cared for when requesting services for family violence.
- All individuals who suffer or have suffered family violence have the right to services and resources that guarantee personal safety and confidentiality.
- All interventions should be carried out in a manner that respects individuals' rights and empowers them to make their own decisions.

Ministry of Health, Costa Rica

TABLE 5-1. TWO ORGANIZATIONAL STRUCTURES FOR THE PLACEMENT OF GBV/FAMILY VIOLENCE CARE PROGRAMS

	Mental Health	Reproductive Health
Advantages	- Increased institutional response in units with specialized resources	- Increased coordination with other programs - Possibility of providing basic care without mental health specialists -More linkages with services for women at high risk
Disadvantages	- Few mental health resources in most of the countries means more difficult to scale up activities - More difficult to coordinate with other programs	- More limited level of response (crisis intervention, basic counseling, and referrals)

LESSONS LEARNED
Inter-programmatic coordination is essential for enabling violence programs to become integrated laterally into key health programs and for ensuring the sustainability of the violence program.

INTER-PROGRAMMATIC COORDINATION IS CRITICAL

Regardless of where the GBV program is located, internal coordination between key programs within the ministries of health that are involved in violence prevention (i.e., mental health, reproductive health, planning, epidemiological surveillance, etc.) is essential.

In most countries, however, with the exception of Costa Rica and Panama, inter-programmatic coordination is weak. This leads to difficulties in implementing norms on violence and inconsistencies in the approach used by different programs within the same ministry. For example, in some ministries each division has a different system for registering information on violence, with the result that the data collected throughout the ministry are not comparable.

WITH NORMS OR WITHOUT THEM ...

Norms and protocols that outline specific responsibilities and tasks that health personnel should carry out with regard to violence is another instrumental step toward securing the uniformity and sustainability of these programs. It is important that all stakeholders, including providers, program managers from other key ministerial divisions, other institutions that coordinate with the health services (forensic medicine institutes, police, etc.), and representatives of nongovernmental organizations, all participate in the development, validation, approval, and implementation of these service polices to ensure that they are both appropriate and feasible to implement.

PAHO's Women, Health, and Development Program provided technical assistance to each of the project countries in the development of national norms and protocols for addressing violence. However, in some countries it has taken years for the norms to be officially approved. To date, norms have been approved in Belize, Costa Rica, Panama, and recently in Nicaragua, whereas in El Salvador and Honduras approval is still pending.

In Guatemala, guidelines for addressing family violence were included in the norms for adolescents and mental health care. However, the scope of these norms is somewhat limited, since they are not included in other key programs, such as reproductive health.

In countries where norms and protocols have not yet been approved, this presents a serious obstacle for the expansion and sustainability of GBV programs. The PAHO program envisioned that the piloted experiences in each country would serve as a laboratory for the development of national policies and norms and would facilitate scaling up the approach in other geographical areas. In the countries

LESSONS LEARNED
In general, having officially approved norms and protocols helps to ensure the quality of care and also facilitates the scaling up of pilot experiences.

Implemented norms and protocols guarantee the quality of care for GBV and family violence in health services. Furthermore, they enable an evaluation of the services.

BOX 5-2. **COSTA RICA'S FAMILY VIOLENCE MODEL APPROACH: KEY ASPECTS**

The goals of family violence intervention are:
- to protect victims of family violence;
- to strengthen the capacity of personnel for decision-making and problem-solving;
- to contribute to healing the effects of violence; and
- to prevent future violence.

Integrated care for family violence should have the following characteristics:
- accessible, continuous, effective, efficient, appropriate, trusting, confidential, secure, quality care that guar-

antees the individual integrity of all those affected;
- care for different types of violence, both within and outside the family, as well as for witnesses of violence;
- a focus on changing the cycle of violence;
- mechanisms for the systematic registration and situation analysis of individuals and families affected by family violence; and
- the ability to accomplish the above components within a permanent monitoring system at a local, regional, and national level.

Ministry of Health, Costa Rica

where GBV norms have been approved, but not been institutionalized, the project has been compelled to continue training health personnel and expanding care and services to new regions in the absence of official guidelines. Health workers consider this to be a significant constraint, as it means that the care for survivors of violence is left up to the discretion of individual staff, without the benefit of a clear protocol detailing how screening, care, and referrals should be performed. Additionally, without protocols in place, it is harder to achieve uniformity in the quality of care or to assess the performance of professionals.

Another challenge that health providers face is high staff turnover in the health sector. This means that even when GBV training has been carried out, new personnel may still lack the necessary experience and skills for providing services to victims of violence. Without this training, safety concerns and confidentiality in the provision of

care may be jeopardized. The existence of norms, protocols, and ongoing supervision would help to minimize these risks.

Nevertheless, in the daily routines of health centers and posts, with or without norms and protocols, health staffs have cared for and continue to care for victims and survivors of family violence. In many places they have found creative solutions to overcome the constraints caused by the absence of norms, in many instances motivated by their own personal commitment and simple desire to help others.

TRAINING HEALTH PERSONNEL
One of the key strategies for raising awareness within the health sector about GBV is to conduct sensitization and technical training for health personnel at all levels.

The review team encountered a great deal of variation in the different countries in terms of the strategies used for training personnel. Some trained all personnel within certain health units. The advantage of this method is that it creates a more supportive environment for GBV issues within the center and motivates all staff, including administrative personnel, to assist in identifying people suffering violence. In other countries, training has been more restricted, such as only to mental health personnel or women's health program staff. Although this approach may result in greater GBV coverage by health centers in general, it is more difficult to achieve impact on the quality of care of people living with violence if only a relatively few staff members within each center are trained. In Honduras, for example, training has been carried out only among the staff of health centers where Family Counseling Centers are located. The main purpose of this training is to encourage staff to refer patients to the counselors.

Given the complexity of GBV and providing care for its victims, there are different levels of training that need to be developed and applied in a strategic manner. In this regard, there is some confusion with respect to the terms **awareness building, training, and specialization.** As a doctor from Nicaragua commented,

". . . Awareness activities lead our staff to the point at which they ask, 'what can we do?' Once we reach this point we can begin training to learn how to actually care for women suffering from family violence."

There is no doubt that the extensive training of health personnel supported by the PAHO project has resulted in considerable increases in the identification of cases, as staff become more confident in their ability to detect violence and offer women support.

In addition to general training of providers, it is also important to include specialized training, such as on forensic medical procedures. Another example is a training conducted by PAHO with the Government of Finland-supported SAREM project in Nicaragua to train psychologists and psychiatrists on how to treat childhood sexual abuse.

Training of trainers is important to ensure sustainability, especially within areas of the ministries of health where staff turnover is constant. In addition to health personnel, consultants from women's NGOs have also been trained as trainers in some instances.

Using effective and tested training materials is important; many are available throughout Latin America and are listed at the end of this book in the GBV Resources Section. In Costa Rica, within the framework of PLANOVI (see Box 4-1.), a set of modules entitled *Feel, Think, and Confront Family Violence* was developed to train staff in identifying and supporting women living with violence. These modules have been used and/or adapted by other Central American countries for training health and other sector personnel. In Guatemala and Peru innovative training packages have been developed that incorporate participatory dynamics adapted to the reality of each country. In Nicaragua many regional health centers have used a training guide for health personnel that was developed by the National Network of Women against Violence.

A significant contribution in all of the countries studied has been the expanded coverage of training to include other social actors: police officers, judges, representatives of women's groups, and schoolteachers. This has been a significant factor in stimulating multisectoral coordination for the project. One example of this work is an integrated "Gender and Family Violence Module" that has been implemented in several schools of public health and nursing schools throughout Central America.

Educational modules on violence have also been created within police academies and the armed forces in some of the countries with the support of the United Nations Latin American Institute for the Prevention of Crime and Treatment of the Delinquent (ILANUD).

Another innovative method for exchanging experiences and promoting "best practices" has been carried out in Estelí, Nicaragua. The health center and anti-violence commission here have created a regional training center where health personnel and community activists from other parts of the country can participate in short internships and receive practical training in GBV care. Perhaps the most valuable aspect of this experience is that the visiting staff spend time not only in the health center, but also in the Women and Children's Police Station and with local NGOs that address violence. As a result, interns learn not only the clinical aspects of care for victims of

violence, but also how to organize community prevention networks. The project has leveraged support from other sources, such as the Swedish Government-supported PROSILAIS project, thereby contributing to the financial sustainability of local networks. This experience could easily be replicated in other health facilities that have specialized care units, such as the Family Counseling Centers in Honduras, or the polyclinic in Barrio Lourdes, El Salvador.

Although a great deal of emphasis has been placed on sensitization and training in the PAHO project, interviews with many health staff indicated that the quality of training was still uneven between countries and between different areas within the same country. There was general agreement that more efforts were needed to develop standardized training curricula that could be adapted for use throughout the Central American subregion.

VIOLENCE INFORMATION AND SURVEILLANCE SYSTEMS: WHAT ISN'T REGISTERED DOESN'T EXIST

Compiling data on violence within the health sector is crucial for demonstrating that gender-based violence is a significant cause of morbidity and mortality. Moreover, data collection provides much-needed insight into potential risk and protective factors, which in turn enable program managers to improve the quality of interventions and policies. As a police captain in Chinandega, Nicaragua, noted,

"With our services and the reports of the *Comisaría* we were able to demonstrate that the lack of personal safety is greater in the home than on the streets."

LESSONS LEARNED

It is important to train all health personnel on the identification of and basic care for women suffering violence. This creates a favorable environment so that individuals may be identified and referred for care by any program within the health center.

Training should include discussions of gender equity and should provide participants not only with technical information, but also with an opportunity to examine their own experiences and beliefs.

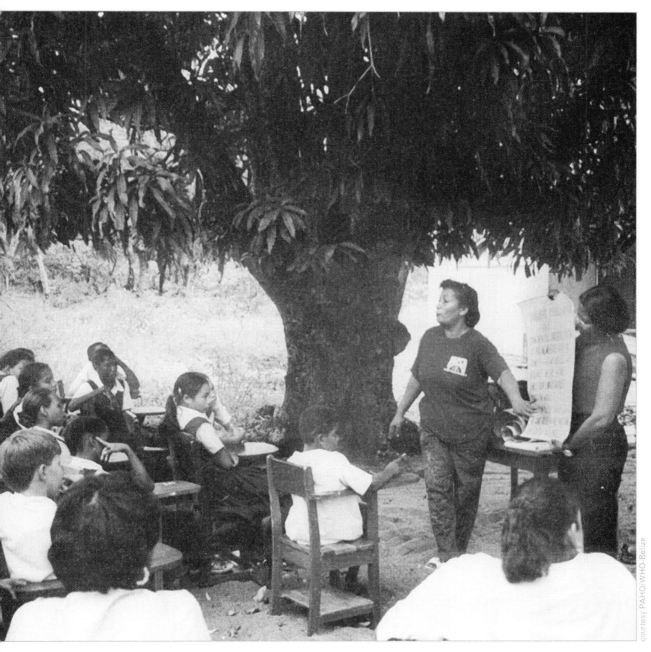

Community development workers
discuss family violence issues with
schoolchildren in a village in Belize.

Over the years, the PAHO project has placed special emphasis on the need to develop violence registration systems within the ministries of health and other sectors for monitoring and guiding interventions.

In all of the project countries there is a commitment to documenting cases of violence even though many challenges in implementation remain. Each of the pilot health centers has set up some kind of registration system for tracking violence, but there is little consistency. The forms used for reporting cases of violence are different among the countries, and even between different regions within some countries (particularly in El Salvador and Nicaragua.)

Providers who attend women and families living with violence are anxious to have an official registration system, in part to increase the legitimacy of addressing the issue, and also so that these activities may be included in personnel performance evaluations. Providers feel pressured by the desire to provide quality care, on the one hand, and the need to fulfill productivity targets demanded by the health services, on the other. Another concern voiced was the need to ensure that once these data are collected, there are also systems in place for their analysis and use.

LESSONS LEARNED

Surveillance systems for violence should consider collecting as a minimum, information identifying the type of violence (i.e., physical, sexual, or emotional), the sex and age of the victim of violence, as well as the age and relationship of the perpetrator to the victim.

In El Salvador and Nicaragua, health workers fill out registration forms and send them to the larger regional offices, where they usually become "stuck", and are not sent on to the national information offices. In Honduras, the forms filled out by the Family Counseling Centers are sent directly to the national mental health department. Because this system bypasses the national statistics office of the Ministry of Health, the data are not included in the national health services statistics or in the epidemiological surveillance system.

This is a generalized problem that affects not only violence programs, but also other health programs such as malaria or dengue. Although there are overall weaknesses in the flow of health information, in the case of violence, the problem appears to be particularly challenging.

National violence surveillance systems have been set up in Belize and Panama, where uniform information is collected in several institutions (i.e., police stations, forensic medicine institutes, health centers, and hospitals, etc.) and analyzed centrally. At the time of the PAHO project review, proposals had been developed for tracking violence in Costa Rica, El Salvador, and Nicaragua, but they had not yet been implemented. One encouraging sign for improved surveillance of violence is the increasing acceptance by statisticians of the 10th International Classification of Diseases, (ICD-10). The ICD-10, currently in use in Belize, Costa Rica, Nicaragua, and Panama, allows for additional codes to be added to the tracking system for injury and disease indicating that violence was a contributing cause. However, in El Salvador and other countries, only primary causes of disease and injury are registered in national statistics, so that even if the ICD-10 codes for violence are used, they may not always appear in national reports.

One problem is that the information resulting from the surveillance systems is not uniform among the countries. Some countries report only on the type of violence without including information on the age and sex of the victim, or the victim's relationship to the offender. In other cases, enormous amounts of information are collected on the characteristics of violent events, as well as on the victims and offenders, but the information is not consolidated or subsequently utilized. In the cases where data are processed, they are often presented in a way that is difficult to interpret (e.g., presenting data on either sex or age of victims but not both, or not distinguishing between characteristics of victims of child sexual abuse and violence by an intimate partner).

As a result, despite the many achievements of PAHO's gender violence project, today it still is not possible to compare statistics among countries in the Central American subregion. A seminar held in 2001 with representatives of the Ministries of Health of the seven nations concluded that the development of a set of key variables and indicators for all countries was an urgent priority. Information identifying the type of violence (i.e., physical, sexual, or emotional), the sex and age of the victim of violence, as well as the age and relationship of the perpetrator to the victim, were considered to constitute basic information that should be included in any registration system.

A final concern by the review team was that in all the countries where there are registration systems, the use of information appears nonetheless to be limited. Although data are collected and sent on to regional and national authorities, there is little analysis of the information or feedback to the health centers for the purpose of local planning.

WITHOUT APPROPRIATE INTERVENTIONS, THERE IS NOTHING TO REGISTER

A major weakness found in several countries included in the review was that the information systems for tracking violence were often developed independently of the norms and protocols for its treatment, resulting in little coordination between the two processes. In some cases, elaborate systems for recording and analyzing violence statistics were put into place even before providers had been trained to identify or treat victims of abuse. Not surprisingly, virtually no cases of violence were detected. The development of information systems in these circumstances can actually be counterproductive, because it gives a false impression that violence is not an important problem. Furthermore, experts have warned that untrained personnel can actually cause additional harm to women by asking about violence in insensitive or victim-blaming ways.

"In order to put the surveillance system into practice, we realized we needed to have specific protocols for caring for violence. Otherwise, there would be no information to register."
—Ministry of Health representative, Belize

UNIFIED INFORMATION SYSTEMS AND MANDATORY REPORTING

In Belize, Guatemala, and Panama, a single registration system is being developed that is intended to be used by professionals from all sectors that come into contact with violence victims, such as the Ministries of Health, law enforcement, the court system, and NGOs. The system also applies to reports by forensic doctors. In Belize, the Ministry of Health is responsible for consoli-

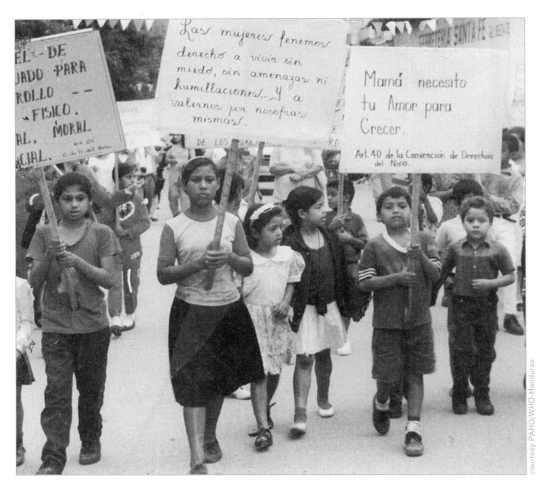

Children are society's least protected members, particularly in matters of family violence.
This group of Honduran children participate in a march to raise awareness about the issue.

dating, processing, and analyzing the information from these sectors and then afterwards reporting it to the other pertinent ministries. In Panama, the information is sent to the Legal Medicine Institute for analysis.

The review team discovered that the difference between filling out a registration form and filing a legal report remains a grey area in many cases. Ideally, the purpose is to collect statistical information, not to set a criminal case into action. However, in Panama and in the proposed system for Guatemala, the information is geared to go automatically to the criminal justice system, equating the completion of the registration form with fil-

ing a criminal report. In both these countries, health providers are required by law to report cases of violence to the legal authorities. In most other Central American countries, health providers are required only to report cases of sexual violence against minors, but not cases of violence against adults.

DOES MANDATORY REPORTING OF VIOLENCE HELP PROTECT WOMEN?

Mandatory reporting presents an ethical dilemma to providers, as it conflicts with a patient's right to confidentiality, as well as with her right to decide how best to deal with her situation, which is one of the guiding principles of the integrated approach. In places where mandatory reporting is required, fines may be imposed on health personnel and other civil servants who do not comply; other ways in which this mandate will be enforced and monitored, however, remain unclear.

Studies in some states in the United States that have mandatory reporting requirements indicate that women are more reluctant to disclose acts of violence if they know this information will be passed on to the police. Providers, likewise, are also less likely to ask about violence if they fear they will be caught up in legal disputes. These concerns were echoed by providers in countries with mandatory reporting laws:

"Victims and survivors are afraid that providers will report the case to the authorities against their will."
—Health provider, Guatemala

"Providers are reluctant to ask about or document violence for fear of the legal consequences of the report, such as becoming involved in court battles, or being a witness, or having their lives placed at risk by threats from the offender."
—Ministry of Health official, Panama

"Even though we have received training in how to fill out the form in the emergency room, health workers do not want to fill it out for fear of the legal repercussions."
—Health provider, Panama

Many ministry of health officials, as well as women's rights activists, expressed the belief that in order to strengthen the health sector's ability to identify and care for victims of violence, it will be necessary to reform the laws regarding mandatory reporting, wherever these exist.

As this chapter has shown, the development and placement of GBV policies within the health sector, the training and sensitization of health personnel, as well as the creation of cohesive and uniform information-gathering and reporting systems capable of being shared by other sectors involved in violence-related issues, are all areas where significant improvements have been marked in the last few years. Despite these achievements, however, significant technical and human challenges remain to be overcome.

In Chapter Six we will take a closer look at what happens behind the doors of the neighborhood health clinic between women and health providers and how their expectations about one another can influence the effectiveness of the care these women receive. ⬱

LESSONS LEARNED
Information and surveillance systems are an essential part of the integrated approach to gender-based violence and should not function independently from the development of services. For the reporting system to work, and before it is implemented, it is important to develop norms and protocols for the detection and care of the affected women and to train providers in their appropriate use. Untrained personnel can actually cause harm to women by asking about violence in insensitive or victim-blaming ways.

Information systems are only valid if the data are used to improve services. Not only is it a waste of resources, but also it is unethical to collect information or carry out active screening for violence with the sole purpose of information-gathering, if no services are offered in return.

Chapter Six

What Happens at the Clinic?

During its evaluation of the PAHO project, the review team found major differences in the quality and types of health services available in different countries, and even in different health facilities within the same pilot communities. However, most providers noted that some combination of the following activities was performed at their centers:

- ✦ SCREENING FOR ABUSE, either through routine questions or upon suspicion that the woman might be a victim of violence;
- ✦ RISK ASSESSMENT, to determine the woman's immediate risk of future violence;
- ✦ APPROPRIATE CARE, including treatment for injuries, addressing reproductive health needs, and crisis intervention;
- ✦ DOCUMENTATION of the violent event and health consequences in the medical charts or on special registration forms;
- ✦ COUNSELING, to provide women with basic information about legal rights and other options and to assist in developing a safety plan, etc.;
- ✦ REFERRALS, either for specialized services within the health system (psychological, forensic medicine, etc.) or to outside institutions (police, child welfare, courts, etc.); and
- ✦ SCHEDULING OF FOLLOW-UP VISITS, to provide continuing support.

This chapter describes the strengths and challenges that providers described in their efforts to integrate care for survivors of violence (i.e., those who had already initiated their "critical path") in ongoing programs.

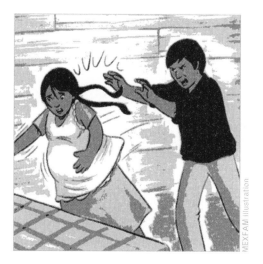

MEXFAM illustration

THE STORY OF ROSITA

In order to facilitate discussions with providers and clients about how women living with violence are treated in the health center, the review team adapted an incomplete story technique first developed by the Mexican Family Planning Foundation (MEXFAM) (Fawcett et al. 1999). In this story, Rosita is the mother of two children who is abused by her husband and feels hopeless about her situation. The story ends when Rosita goes to the health center for a routine visit and the nurse asks her whether she has ever been mistreated by her husband. The exercise is carried out in a group setting, and the participants are asked to imagine how the story ends through a discussion of the following questions:

→ What will Rosita tell the nurse when she asks her questions about violence?

→ How will Rosita feel when she is asked about violence?

→ How does the nurse feel about asking Rosita about her family life?

→ What will happen to Rosita if she admits what is happening to her at home?

→ What type of help would be most useful to her?

→ Do you think she will receive this help at the health center?

→ Do you think Rosita's situation is common among women in this community?

These questions were used to introduce a more focussed discussion on the type and quality of services offered to women in Rosita's situation at the participants' health center.

IDENTIFYING WOMEN LIVING WITH VIOLENCE

The approaches that providers use to identify women living with violence vary greatly among the Central American countries studied and even among clinics within the same country. The various approaches may be categorized in the following way:

→ **not asking any direct screening questions.** Most providers in Guatemala did not ask women directly about violence, even when there were signs of abuse, but if women disclosed violence on their own the providers would try to offer support. In Guatemala the GBV norms are part of the national mental health program, and there is no official policy on screening, so identification of violence is largely left to the discretion of the individual provider. International experience has shown that this is generally not an effective strategy for identifying survivors of violence.

→ **universal screening** refers to a policy of asking all women about violence in every program and on every visit. The Ministry of Health and the Social Security Institute of Costa Rica have proposed implementing universal screening in their GBV norms. This system is the most far-reaching; however, it is also the most costly and difficult to implement, particularly in low resource settings.

→ **asking whenever violence is suspected.** This approach was commonly used in

El Salvador and Honduras. It can be a cost-effective way to identify women, but only if the staff are well-trained and motivated.

➤ **integrating GBV screening and services into selected "sentinel" programs**. This means carrying out routine screening in certain priority areas where abused women are more likely to be identified (for example, in emergency services or mental health programs) or in areas where identifying a history of violence is most likely to improve the overall quality of services (i.e., prenatal care, STIs, family planning, etc.). This approach was adopted in Nicaragua's GBV norms; however, it has not yet been fully implemented.

Since these GBV programs are still relatively new, it is perhaps still too early to assess the most successful approaches for identifying women living with violence. Nevertheless, it seems evident that the first two options are less likely to be as effective as the latter two. Experience has demonstrated that programs without a screening policy identify only a fraction of those women requiring assistance. On the other hand, it is not feasible to implement universal screening in the majority of

Central American health services, given the scarcity of qualified resources and time pressures experienced by health personnel.

However, a mixed strategy consisting of screening all women with signs of abuse in all programs and performing routine screening of all women in certain "sentinel" programs might be an effective compromise. This approach would allow providers to optimize resources by targeting women who are at greatest risk for abuse. Moreover, integrating screening and care for survivors of violence into reproductive and mental health programs could contribute to enhancing the quality of care in these programs, as well.

"WOMEN ARE WAITING FOR SOMEONE TO KNOCK ON THEIR DOOR..."
Results of a Screening Exercise for Violence

To date, most experiences with screening have taken place in Canada, Europe, and the United States, where conditions are generally quite different from those of health services in low resource settings. In order to assess the feasibility of introducing a policy of screening for violence, PAHO conducted a study in four Central American countries between 1999 and 2000. The purpose of the study was to determine the acceptability of routine screening among health workers and clients and whether the use of a screening instrument would enhance identification of violence in the clinical setting. At each site, all personnel, including administrative staff, were sensitized about GBV. Providers were trained in the use of a screening instrument that consisted of three questions about recent experiences with physical or emotional violence involving a partner. During a one-to-three-month period, staff used the instrument to screen all women between the ages of 15–44 who came to the health center for any reason. On average, the questions took about three minutes to ask. Subsequent interviews with the health workers, as well

> ## LESSONS LEARNED
> It is not enough to simply wait for women to disclose violence on their own. Experience has shown that many women are willing to talk about violence, but it is usually necessary for health personnel to take the initiative and open the discussion.
>
> Screening for violence may be performed in any area of health services. The most important requisites for an effective screening program are privacy, trained and empathetic staff, and the ability to listen and offer some basic counseling.

> **BOX 6-1. TYPES OF COMPLAINTS LEADING PROVIDERS TO SUSPECT VIOLENCE**
>
> - Anxiety
> - Allergies
> - Gastritis
> - Colitis
> - Migraines
> - Bumps/bruises or unexplained injuries
> - High blood pressure
> - Learning problems in children
> - Sexually transmitted infections
> - Termination of medical visits
>
> *Statements by health personnel and clients in El Salvador*

they feel comfortable discussing the issue. Discussions with providers in Barrio Lourdes, El Salvador, about the screening experience confirmed this view:

"Sometimes we have to ask the question on a couple of visits. Maybe the first time it comes as a shock, but by the second time she begins to trust us."

"A woman's reaction depends on the level of trust that we provide. When you first start this process, it feels horrible, but not anymore. The most important thing is to listen to her, and not write at the same time, but rather give her your full attention so that you don't lose her."

> **BOX 6-2. IPPF'S SCREENING TOOL FOR GBV**
>
> - Have you ever felt hurt emotionally or psychologically by your partner or another person important to you?
> - Has your partner or another person important to you ever caused you physical harm?
> - Were you ever forced to have sexual contact or intercourse?
> - When you were a child, were you ever touched in a way that made you feel uncomfortable?
> - Do you feel safe returning to your home tonight?
>
> *(The full instrument is available at the IPPF Web site at www.ippfwhr.org.)*

as their clients, revealed that both groups felt comfortable with the questions.

The study revealed that between 12% and 54% of all clients disclosed experiences of recent physical or emotional partner violence. Reproductive health services generally identified the highest proportion of cases of violence. Surprisingly, the number of abused women identified varied greatly among the different health centers, sometimes even among those within the same communities.

The variation in disclosure rates is likely due to a number of factors. International research has shown that women's willingness to disclose violence depends on many factors beyond the specific wording of questions. For example, the skill and interest of personnel asking the questions, the level of awareness among the general population, the existence of referral services, and whether the screening is performed in privacy are all factors that may influence disclosure. Some studies have found that it may be necessary to ask women about violence on more than one occasion before

Most of the providers who participated in the screening exercise found it to be an eye-opening experience. It revealed to them the extent to which violence can contribute to a woman's complaint, even though she may not mention it as the purpose of her visit. This understanding has changed the way many health workers view their work. For example, as one physical therapist from the Barrio Lourdes clinic in San Salvador explained,

"I used to treat women with muscle spasms all the time, and I never asked them any questions. Then I started to realize that many of these cases were due to violence."

A psychologist from the same clinic added,

"The textbooks tell me how to treat depression, but now we have begun to change our diagnoses. We see that a patient may suffer from depression; however, it is secondary to the domestic violence problem. With this insight we can find a better approach to help her."

A second valuable insight from the screening exercise was that, contrary to initial expectations, women were not only willing to talk about their experiences of violence, but often deeply grateful for the opportunity to tell their stories.

LESSONS LEARNED

Encouraging health personnel to screen women for violence in their regular practice can be an excellent exercise for raising general awareness and helping personnel to become more confident in treating cases of violence. Ideally, the screening instrument should include questions on physical, emotional, and sexual violence, and should include experiences that have occurred at any point in the client's lifetime, as well as the most recent experiences. In prenatal clinics, the screening instrument should also ask about violence during the current pregnancy.

After completing the exercise, it is important to implement and monitor a permanent policy for screening and care of the survivors in order to maintain the achievements of the initial exercise.

"Women are waiting for someone to knock on their door; some of them have been waiting for many years. . . . They are grateful for the opportunity to unload their burden."
—Nurse, El Salvador

Finally, the experience demonstrated the importance of involving all staff in the training on GBV. In one health center in El Salvador, the medical director noted that he had initially been skeptical about the screening exercise, as he had never had a woman disclose instances of violence in a medical visit before. After participating in the exercise, he became an enthusiastic convert: "I challenged myself to become more alert about possible cases [of violence], and I realized that it was not as difficult as I had thought." Not only does this physician now routinely ask his patients about violence, but he also obtained funds from the Ministry of Health to build an additional space in the health center so that women could talk to counselors in privacy. Box 6-3. illustrates several informal screening techniques used by health workers in a variety of health programs.

Many other programs have also found that the routine use of a short screening tool can greatly increase identification rates for violence (McFarlane et al. 1991; Feldhaus et al. 1997). IPPF has carried out a program in three Latin American affiliates (the Dominican Republic, Peru, and Venezuela) to integrate services for GBV into existing reproductive health programs. The providers found that by introducing a five-question screening tool into the client history-taking for all new clients, identification of women who had suffered GBV increased to 38% of all new clients, compared with only 7% when providers asked questions at their own discretion (Guedes et al. 2002).

Among the PAHO project communities, the screening experience gave staff confidence in their own abilities and motivated them to

---

BOX 6-3. INDIRECT WAYS TO START A CONVERSATION ABOUT VIOLENCE

In family planning clinics

- *We ask if her husband agrees with family planning. If she says no, then we know that there are problems.*
- *In the exam I ask her how she feels about family planning and what would happen if he were aware. I let her know that her body belongs to her, even if her husband doesn't want to practice family planning.*
- *You might become aware of [violence] because of a husband's jealousy and control. For example, sometimes they will say that they don't practice family planning "because he doesn't want anyone to see me."*

In cancer prevention programs

- *Sometimes while taking a Pap smear, I'll see older women with injuries, dryness, and bruises from forced sex.*
- *When I see bruises I ask, "What happened here?" The women start to cry and say that they do not go for their routine exams because their husbands keep them locked in the house.*

In child wellness programs

- *I don't ask directly [about violence] because women might become afraid. I say, "Are there problems in the house? How does the father get along with the children? How do the children get along with each other?" Sometimes there is nothing wrong with the child but I use it as a ploy to talk with the mother.*

During dermatology consultations

- *After several visits for a chronic allergy on her hands, I asked her if she was having problems at home, and that is when she started to cry.*

Statements from health workers in El Salvador

---

continue asking about violence. However, the exercise alone was not sufficient to change providers' behavior. In the centers where new policies on screening and care for survivors of violence were not implemented and monitored with strong, sustained leadership and support from management, some momentum was eventually lost over time. In these centers staff admitted that they no longer asked women about violence on a routine basis. Similar results were found in a study of a U.S. emergency room, where screening protocols had been instituted with great success. However, a few years later, it was found that levels of detection had fallen back to the initial levels, due to the lack of monitoring and follow-up support to staff (McLeer et al. 1989). These experiences underscore the importance of using a "systems" approach to integrating violence into health programs, including institutional policies and protocols for identifying and treating victims of abuse.

IF SHE SAYS YES, THEN WHAT?

A concern that has frequently been voiced with regard to GBV screening programs is that too much emphasis is placed on screening as an end in itself, without enough consideration of what happens next. Some critics question whether it is even ethical to screen for violence if there is not a program in place and services to refer women to once they disclose violence (García-Moreno 2002). This concern is echoed by health workers who fear that if a patient discloses violence, it will open up a "Pandora's Box" of problems that they will not know how to respond to (Sugg and Inui 1992). This is a particular concern in low resource settings, where there may be few or no places to which to refer women suffering abuse. Others argue that asking about violence is, in itself, an intervention, by signaling to women that violence is unacceptable and that it can affect their health. One of the primary aims of this review was to hear what providers and women clients felt were the most important strengths of the GBV programs, in addition to their more visible weaknesses.

In each country there was at least one pilot health center that had one or more specialists (either social workers, psychologists, and/or psychiatrists) who had been trained to work with survivors of abuse. In Honduras, women who are identified as abuse survivors by health providers are referred directly to the Family Counseling Centers (FCC), which have been established in each of the country's 13 health dis-

tricts. Women receive individual or group counseling at the FCC, and if necessary, may be referred to the police, child welfare department, or the human rights commission for additional help. Some of the FCC clients who were interviewed had been in individual therapy for more than one year and expressed great satisfaction with the support they had received. However, this model of care is neither feasible nor cost-effective in many low resource settings where counseling services of this type are either scarce or nonexistent.

An alternative strategy that has worked well in these settings is to designate one or more staff as GBV counselors. For example, at the Chintúc health center in El Salvador, four nurses were trained to provide crisis intervention and basic counseling. On each shift the supervising nurse makes sure that there is at least one trained counselor available. This strategy ensures that providers have backup resources whenever they identify a woman that needs help. Furthermore, the center has established prioritized care for survivors of violence so that they may be treated immediately without having to wait in line. To ensure privacy, some centers, such as Chintúc in El Salvador and the Estelí health center in Nicaragua, have designated special rooms that can be used for counseling. In other cases, administrative offices are used to ensure privacy.

This approach provides effective basic support for women in the absence of specialized services. Providers are more likely to screen for violence when they know that backup support is available to them. Counselors are able to provide primary crisis intervention and counseling, as well as basic information on existing laws and services and how to develop a safety plan. When other services in the community are available, such as women's centers, the counselors give referrals and often coordinate care with these centers.

LESSONS LEARNED

It is not necessary to have specialized personnel in mental health to provide quality care for victims of violence.

What is essential is to motivate and train staff and to organize services so that women that need support receive treatment with a human quality and in a timely manner.

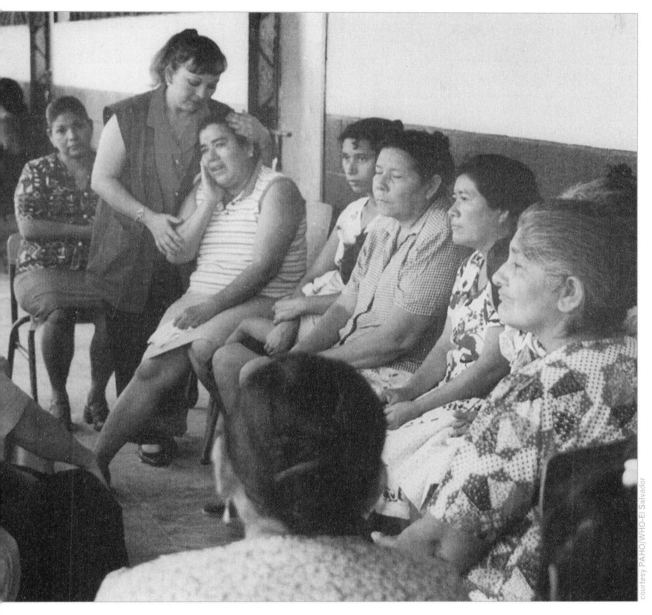

Women's support and self-help groups,
such as this one in El Salvador, give
women the opportunity to help each
other and to realize that others care
and they are not the only ones that suffer
from violence. The bonds of solidarity
that are formed can empower women
to transform their situations and end
the violence through mutual support.

One limitation of this approach that was noted is the lack of capacity for providing follow-up to women. As one nurse at the Chintúc health center explained, at times, if the health personnel are particularly concerned about a woman, they will develop creative mechanisms that will enable them to check on clients:

"Sometimes we visit her at home, but cover it up with other activities such as vaccination."

Unfortunately, however, most providers reported having little time or resources for follow-up activities and acknowledged that it is not uncommon for them to lose track of clients who stop coming to the clinic or simply never return after the initial visit. At the Barrio Lourdes Polyclinic in El Salvador, which specializes in community mental health care, a similar basic approach to care is used. All personnel were sensitized in GBV and trained to screen women whenever they suspect abuse. In addition, several staff members were given additional training to provide emotional support and to facilitate support groups for survivors. Because of the center's close ties to the community in general, it has been successful in providing long-term follow-up and support to women, including individual psychological care and the development of support groups for survivors. The GBV counselors come from a variety of disciplines, including physical therapy, special education, and nursing. The center's psychologist provides supervision, guidance, and emotional support to the violence counselors and receives referrals from them in cases that require specialized care.

When asked what kind of professional profile they thought was most suitable for a GBV counselor, the staff at Barrio Lourdes noted almost unanimously that a person's profession or gender was less important than personal motivation, and this explained why their own counselors had such diverse backgrounds.

LISTENING IS KEY

"I tell her, if she wants to cry, she should cry; if she wants to talk, she should talk. . . . When she calms down, we help her to think about what she will do and what options she has."
—Nurse, El Salvador

When a woman decides to talk to her provider about violence it may be the first time that she has ever disclosed her situation to anyone, including her own family. Therefore, providers have an enormous responsibility to ensure that, at the very least, women are treated with respect and compassion and that they do not contribute to "revictimizing" patients through indifference or by making women feel that they are to blame for their situations. (More information about how providers can help women living with violence is provided in Box 6-4.) Health workers stressed the importance of listening and allowing women to tell their stories without rushing them. A Salvadoran doctor, who acknowledged that he used to get impatient if a patient started to cry in his office, confessed that, after the training, his attitude changed:

"Now, I let her get out the last tear because I know this helps her. I refer her for help afterwards, but when she leaves she already feels relieved."

The providers felt that what women most wanted was an opportunity to talk, without fear of being judged.

"Just listening to them lifts a huge weight off of their shoulders. That in itself is a lot."
—Nurse, El Salvador

"I like to make women laugh, because sometimes it is important to see the positive side of things. I am not satisfied unless she leaves smiling."
—Doctor, El Salvador

"Sometimes women come to us, not expecting us to solve their problems, but rather just to be listened to . . . what they hope for is some advice."
—Doctor, El Salvador

In addition to listening to women, providers can help women assess whether they or their children are in immediate danger. There are several instruments that have been used internationally for this purpose, such as the Danger Assessment Screen (Campbell 1995). The IPPF program asks all women: "Do you feel safe returning home tonight?" (Guedes et al. 2002). Depending on her response, providers can help her to review options and to develop a safety plan to protect her and her family in the future (Box 6-6. gives an example of how to develop a safety plan).

As the following account from a Guatemalan nurse suggests, providers may have only one opportunity to intervene:

"Once I treated a woman who came for a headache. When I asked her, it turned out that her husband had been sharpening his machete for the last three days, saying that he was going to kill her. She had spent the whole time wondering where he would cut her first and that was how she got the headache. We had to develop a safety plan with her right then because she said she would not be able to return."

Another lesson that many providers expressed is that it is impossible to provide quality care, particularly in the case of reproductive health services, unless they take into account the specific needs of women living with violence. For example, a nurse from El Salvador explained how important it is to know whether a woman is suffering violence before advising her about family planning methods, as many abused women are not able to use contraceptives to avoid unwanted pregnancies without their husbands' permission:

"We try to help abused women who want to use family planning, but our problem is that we can't provide monthly injections, which is the only method that can be concealed. If a woman uses an IUD her husband might feel it, and the pills are dangerous because he might find them. If she uses the three-month injection method she won't get her period and her husband might become suspicious. Sometimes we tell them to have their friends keep their pills so that the husband won't notice."

Both providers and women agreed that the most helpful messages that providers can give to survivors of violence is that violence is wrong and that it is not her fault.

"I tell her, 'What is happening to you has a name: it is called family violence.' Then I give her a brochure and ask her to come back when she is convinced that she needs help."
—Nurse, El Salvador

"Oftentimes they feel guilty. I tell them that nothing justifies this treatment. . . . I try to show them that violence is not normal; that they have rights." —Nurse, El Salvador

"I can't let her leave while she is still crying, as this will scare off the other patients; I want her to leave smiling; I tell her how brave she is."
—Doctor, El Salvador

For a woman who has been living with overwhelming shame and guilt for many years, this message can be nothing short of life-transforming. As one Honduran woman who had even contemplated suicide as her "only way out" noted, the care and support of health workers had, in fact, saved her life and taught her how to accept and respect herself.

BOX 6-4. HOW CAN HEALTH WORKERS BEST SUPPORT WOMEN LIVING WITH ABUSE?

Health workers often feel that there is little they can do when a woman discloses abuse. But what providers say and do can have an important influence on a woman's course of action (McCauley et al. 1998; Gerbert et al. 1999). The act of asking questions about violence can let women know that providers consider violence to be an important medical problem and not the client's fault. As one Latin American woman said: "The doctor helped me feel better by saying that I didn't deserve this treatment, and he helped me make a plan to leave the house the next time my husband came home drunk," (Sagot 2000).

Women in the United States also emphasize the power of validation, noting that it provided "relief," and "comfort," and "planted a seed," and "started the wheels turning" toward changing their perception of their own situation (Gerbert et al. 1999). Some of the ways in which health workers can promote healing for women living with violence are described in the "Empowerment Wheel" used in violence prevention training (see Box 6-5.).

Even if an abused woman does not disclose the violence on a first visit, asking about it shows that the clinician cares and may encourage her to talk about it on a later visit. While health workers ideally should coordinate their actions with other community-based services, such as local women's groups, providers can take several useful steps during the initial clinic visit (Parker and Campbell 1991; Warshaw and Ganley 1998).

1. Assess for immediate danger. Find out whether the woman feels that she or her children are in immediate danger. If so, help her consider various courses of action. Is there a friend or relative who can help her? If there is a women's shelter or crisis center in the area, offer to make the contact for her. Some hospitals and clinics have adopted explicit policies allowing abused women to be admitted overnight if it is unsafe for them to return home (Josiah 1998; Leye et al. 1999). Leaving a violent partner temporarily does not necessarily end the violence, however. The most dangerous moment for a woman with an abusive partner is often immediately after she leaves or announces her decision to leave a relationship (Campbell 1995).

2. Provide appropriate care. For women who have suffered sexual assault, appropriate care may include providing emergency contraception and presumptive treatment for gonorrhea, syphilis, or other locally prevalent STIs. Unless clearly necessary, clinicians should avoid prescribing tranquilizers and mood-altering drugs to women who are living with an abusive partner since these may impair their ability to predict and react to their partners' attacks.

3. Document the woman's condition.
Few providers adequately document cases of abuse against women. In Johannesburg, South Africa, a review found that in 78% of cases of abuse providers had not recorded the identity of the perpetrator. Clinical records included such graphic but general descriptions as "chopped with an axe" or "stabbed with a knife" (Motsei and the Centre for Health Policy 1993). Careful documentation of a woman's symptoms or injuries, as well as of her history of abuse, are helpful for future medical follow-up. Documentation is also important in the event that she decides to press charges against the abuser or to seek custody of the children. Documentation should be as thorough as possible and clearly state the identity of the offender and his or her relationship to the victim.

4. Develop a safety plan. Although women cannot prevent violence from recurring and they may not be ready to report their partner to the police, there are ways that they can protect themselves and their children. These include keeping a bag packed with important documents, keys, and a change of clothes, or developing a signal to let children know when they need to seek help from neighbors. Health care providers should review a sample safety plan with the woman and decide together which actions may help in her situation (see Box 6-6.). Sample safety plans can also be taped to the walls of the clinic's

restroom and examining room, where women may read them in privacy and without embarrassment.

5. Inform the woman of her rights.
When a woman takes the step of disclosing her situation, it is crucial that medical practitioners reaffirm that the violence is not her fault and that no one deserves to be beaten or raped. The penal codes of most countries criminalize rape and physical assault, even if specific laws against domestic violence do not exist. Medical staff should find out what legal protections exist for victims of abuse and where women and children can turn for genuine help in enforcing their rights.

6. Refer the woman to other community resources. Health care providers can help victims of abuse through early detection and by referring them to available local resources. The needs of victims generally extend beyond what the health sector alone is able to provide. Therefore it is essential that health care providers know in advance what other resources are available to help victims of abuse. It is especially useful for health workers to meet personally with others who provide services for victims of violence because providers will be more likely to refer a woman to someone whom they know when there is a face behind the name.

From: Heise, Ellsberg, and Goettemoeller 1999)

BOX 6-5. GENDER-BASED VIOLENCE: ARE HEALTH WORKERS PART OF THE PROBLEM?

ESCALATING DANGER

Violating confidentiality...
Interviewing in front of family. Telling colleagues issues discussed in confidence without her consent. Calling the police without her consent.

Normalizing victimization...
Failing to respond to her disclosure of abuse. Acceptance of intimidation as normal in relationships. Belief that abuse is the outcome of noncompliance with patriarchy.

Trivializing and minimizing the abuse...
Not taking the danger she feels seriously. Assuming that if she's lived with it for years, it's not serious. Insisting that the family be kept together.

HEALTH WORKERS CAN HURT WOMEN BY...

Ignoring her need for safety...
Failing to recognize her sense of danger. Not asking: "Is it safe to go home? Do you have a place you could go if the situation escalates?"

Blaming the victim...
Asking what she did to provoke the abuse. Focusing on her as the problem: "Why don't you just leave? Why do you put up with it? Why do you let him do that to you?"

Not respecting her autonomy...
"Prescribing" divorce, sedative medicines, going to a shelter, couples counseling, or law enforcement involvement. Punishing the patient for not taking a doctor's advice.

INCREASED ENTRAPMENT

...OR ARE HEALTH WORKERS PART OF THE SOLUTION?

EMPOWERMENT

Respecting her confidentiality...
All discussion must occur in private, without other family members present. This is essential to building trust and ensuring her safety.

Promoting access to community services...
Know and share resources in your community: a hotline, a shelter for battered women, counselors, support groups, legal services.

Believing and validating her experiences...
Listen to her and believe her. Acknowledge her feelings and let her know she is not alone.

HEALTH WORKERS CAN HELP WOMEN BY...

Helping her plan for future safety...
What has she tried in the past to keep herself and her children safe? Is it working? Does she have a place to go if she needs to escape?

Acknowledging the injustice...
The violence perpetrated against her is not her fault. No one deserves to be abused.

Respecting her autonomy...
Respect her right to make decisions about her situation, when she is ready. She knows what is best under the circumstances.

EMPOWERMENT

The Medical and Power Wheel, developed by the Domestic Violence Project, Inc. Kenosha, Wisconsin, U.S.A.

BOX 6-6. DEVELOPING A SAFETY PLAN

Health care providers can help women protect themselves from intimate partner violence, even if the women may not be ready to leave home or report abusive partners to authorities. When clients have a personal safety plan, they are better able to deal with violent situations. Providers can review these points below to help each woman develop her own personal safety plan:

- Identify one or more neighbors you can tell about the violence, and ask them to seek help if they hear a disturbance in your home.
- If an argument seems unavoidable, try to have it in a room or an area that you can leave easily.
- Stay away from any room where weapons might be available.
- Practice how to get out of your home safely. Identify which doors, windows, elevator, or stairwell would be best.
- Have a packed bag ready, containing spare keys, money, important documents, and clothes. Keep it at the home of a relative or friend, in case you need to leave your own home in a hurry.
- Devise a code word to use with your children, family, friends, and neighbors when you need emergency help or want them to call the police.
- Decide where you will go if you have to leave home, and have a plan to get there.
- Use your instincts and judgment. If the situation is dangerous, consider giving the abuser what he is demanding to calm him down. You have the right to protect yourself and your children.
- Remember: you do not deserve to be hit or threatened.

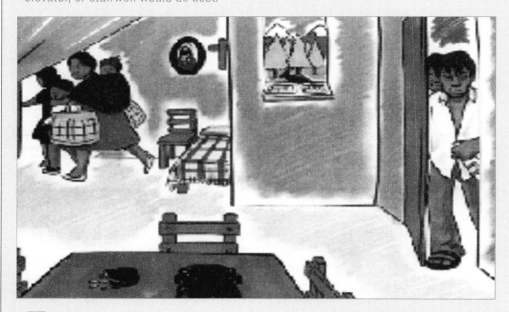

Adapted from Buel 1995 in Heise et al. 1999
MEXFAM illustration

"IN THE BEGINNING I USED TO CRY ALONG WITH THEM. . . ."
Health Providers Also Need Emotional Support

One of the themes that emerged in the assessment was how deeply providers were affected by caring for survivors of violence. "We've all had moments when the floor moves beneath us," acknowledged a Salvadoran psychologist. Many mentioned effects ranging from being exhausted emotionally to fear of retaliation by aggressors

to frustration with women "who do not follow our advice." The stories of rape, humiliation, injuries, and death threats leave physical and emotional scars on those who listen to them. As one study pointed out, "trauma is contagious," and can manifest itself in emotional problems: depression, anxiety, fear, or insensitivity to the pain of those suffering. It can also be exhibited in physical symptoms such as chronic exhaustion, chronic pain, gastric problems, or changes in sleeping patterns (Claramunt 1999). Some of the reactions of providers are described in Box 6-7.

One issue that is often hard for providers to accept is that they may not be able to "fix" a woman's problem. What is even more challenging is that, as the Critical Path study showed, the woman may decide not to follow the provider's advice or to take actions that providers don't understand. This can be frustrating, particularly for doctors, who are trained to measure success by patient compliance and whether or not an illness is cured. In a discussion group with providers in Barrio Lourdes in El Salvador, several nurses acknowledged that this was often a challenge:

"Sometimes I feel angry with her; I wish I could make her understand."

"Sometimes we are overwhelmed with our patients' problems. We want to help them to wake up and react. We would like to see them move out of the situation because the way out is clear to us."

"Sometimes I wish I could make the decision for her, or tell her to leave him. But you can't tell someone what to do."

In some places, threats to their own physical safety must be added to the list of challenges that providers face. In one case described by Guatemalan providers, masked men

---

BOX 6-7. PROVIDERS' RESPONSES TO VIOLENCE

"In the beginning, I used to cry along with them. . . ."

"I feel as though asking them questions is like revictimizing them."

"Sometimes I feel powerless and I don't know how to help her. . . ."

"The day before my vacation my last patient arrived with bruises, and her daughter had strangulation marks on her neck. I got a lump in my throat and forgot everything I had been taught. I went home praying to God that he wouldn't kill her while I was away."

"Three or four months after coming here and before I received training I had a case of a woman who had been beaten by her husband and raped by her older brother when she was 7 years old. Her situation really got to me, and I wasn't able to sleep for several days."

Statements by health workers from Barrio Lourdes, El Salvador

LESSONS LEARNED
Emotional support is essential for health providers who care for survivors of violence.

Activities to ensure support for personnel should be included in norms and implemented at the local level.

attacked an NGO that managed a shelter for survivors of violence and raped several members of its team. The shelter eventually closed down. Naturally, these experiences create fear among personnel. As one Guatemalan nurse admitted:

"Sometimes you feel afraid because a woman might reveal to her husband what you talked about during the exam."

Another nurse recalled treating a woman while her armed husband stalked outside the center looking for her:

"I felt unsafe; I thought: when is this man going to come looking for me?"

A psychologist from Guatemala City also noted:

"Once you get involved in this, you know you are on your own, as there is no protection for us. I've learned that it's better just to relax, because if you become afraid, you won't be able to go on."

Although caring for women suffering from violence is very draining, many providers also mentioned positive experiences in their personal and professional lives. Many observed that the awareness workshops had helped them to overcome their own experiences of violence and fears and to strengthen bonds with their other colleagues. As two providers in El Salvador observed:

"This health unit works very well. It is like wiping away the dirt to see yourself in the mirror."

"The awareness helped us get to know one another better and to have more consideration for each other."

Emotional support for providers should be considered as an essential component of any program to address GBV. Emotional support refers to any kind of activity that

BOX 6-8. **TAKING CARE OF OURSELVES: SUGGESTIONS FOR PRACTICING SELF-HELP FOR PROVIDERS WORKING WITH GBV**

- **Getting to know our own history:** When we work in the field of family violence, the process of self-help begins by healing the wounds of personal abuse, when these exist.
- **Taking care of our bodies:**
  - Deep breathing exercises
  - Physical exercise
  - Eating well
  - Getting enough sleep and resting
  - Practices that aid relaxation and healing and provide energy, such as aromatherapy, bioenergetics, and music therapy
- **Transforming our thoughts:**
  - Flexibility
  - Optimism
  - Understanding and empathy
  - Relativism in evaluating problems, viewing them as an opportunity to learn and to change old habits
  - Taking responsibility for our decisions and actions
  - Thinking in the present tense
- **Staying in touch with our feelings**
- **Reviewing what we have accomplished every day**

From: Claramunt 1999

helps to reduce stress and anxiety, including recreation or sessions for discussing the feelings and emotions that result from their professional responsibilities. PAHO has developed a guide for the emotional support for providers (Claramunt 1999). Nevertheless, only one of the centers visited by the review team mentioned holding occasional support activities for providers. On the other hand, all of the providers agreed that more attention should be given to this issue in the future.

"THIS CENTER IS DIFFERENT; IT IS WARMER"

Reflections on 10 Years of Experience

Despite the many difficulties that they have faced, health providers who work with GBV expressed a great deal of pride and satisfaction in their accomplishments (see Box 6-10. for a list of topics most frequently mentioned). Most importantly, providers felt that dealing with violence had improved the quality of care in the center.

BOX 6-9. FUTURE STEPS FOR STRENGTHENING GBV WORK

- Develop a protocol for screening and care for victims
- Create indicators for evaluating the program
- Design a better registration system
- Prepare budget for evaluation
- Incorporate more follow-up training
- Spread the program to other centers: "others should be following our example—it's not rocket science"
- Assign special rooms for talking to women
- Receive more training in legal issues
- Ensure more emotional support for staff: "we need a space to talk about what has happened"
- Include a psychologist or psychiatrist for referrals

Statements by health workers at Chintúc Health Center, Apopa, El Salvador

---

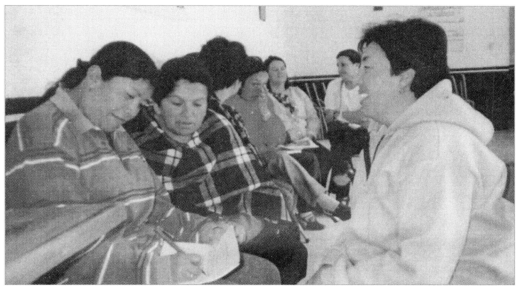

courtesy PAHO/WHO-Ecuador

Women respond most positively to community staff who have effective personal skills and show true interest in the women and their situations.

BOX 6-10. CARE FOR VICTIMS OF FAMILY VIOLENCE: STRENGTHS AND CONSTRAINTS

Within the health services
- Recognition of violence as a health problem with many different possible physical and mental manifestations
- Greater credibility and respect among health personnel
- Overall improvements in the quality of care
- Changes in the providers' attitudes
- Having physical spaces to care for victims in the health center
- Having more integrated services for family violence
- Having basic tools for addressing violence
- Having financial support from PAHO

In relation to the community
- Feeling a greater closeness to the community now
- Better coordination with the police and district attorney's offices
- Increased client demand for services
- Increased community awareness about violence

At a personal level
- Satisfaction from being able to help others
- Acquiring new skills and knowledge

Within the health services
- Lack of approval and dissemination of norms and protocols
- High staff turnover
- Work overload
- Not having enough time to attend to clients' needs adequately
- Lack of paper supplies
- Limitations in the registry/ epidemiological surveillance systems
- Lack of interest by some staff in the subject
- Lack of a permanent plan for communication and information
- Lack of self-care activities
- Lack of adequate spaces for guaranteeing privacy
- Lack of financial resources for training and follow-up of cases
- Lack of support from some clinic directors
- Incomplete transfer of knowledge at times to others following training by some staff
- Lack of trained mental health resources
- Lack of training materials
- Lack of informational/promotional materials (posters, pamphlets, etc.)

At a community level
- The attitudes of some clients (not accepting that they live with violence, unwilling to accept help)
- Problems in coordination and referrals
- Problems with the justice system (laws are not enforced)

———
Statements by health workers in Estelí, Nicaragua

"People tell us that this center is different;
it is warmer. . . .They come here because
we listen to them. . . ."
—Nurse, El Salvador

Another achievement mentioned by several
providers was a transformation in the role
of health workers and particularly the
empowerment of nurses:

"Nurses have become aware of this issue.They
understand that their job is more than taking someone's blood pressure or drawing blood. Breaking
out of the traditional mold in every area was a big
development."
—Nurse, El Salvador

In terms of the barriers faced by personnel
with respect to violence-related care,
the majority have to do with the work
environment (lack of privacy, time pressures,
productivity) or with administrative concerns,
such as the lack of senior-level support.
The lack of accepted norms and information
and epidemiological surveillance systems
was a constraint mentioned by many of
the providers. Better reporting of cases of
violence registered within the health system
would help justify the time that is devoted
to caring for survivors, as well as demonstrate more definitively that violence is an
important health problem.

Both providers at the clinic level and
national program coordinators agreed that
the major challenge facing them is to use
the wealth of lessons gained from the pilot
experiences in order to scale up to national
programs while ensuring the sustainability
of the existing programs. In some countries,
particularly in Costa Rica and Panama,
considerable progress has been made in
institutionalizing the GBV program through
national policies and budgetary allocations.
In El Salvador and Nicaragua, PAHO and
the Ministries of Health have been able

to extend the coverage of the program
by leveraging resources from other
international projects, such as the Swedish
Government-supported health reform
programs in both countries.

Perhaps the greatest source of pride
mentioned by health providers was the
improvement in their relationship with the
community. Providers felt great satisfaction
in the belief that they were contributing,
not only to improving the lives of individual
women and families, but also to transforming
the way community members view violence
in general:

"We are closer to the community now. People go
to the health centers more often. Our clients have
become our best promoters."
—Nurse, El Salvador

"People are familiar with the laws and know
that they are protected. Nowadays women are
no longer afraid to report violence."
—Nurse, El Salvador

In Chapter Seven, we will go beyond the
clinical setting to the community at large,
where we will see how local resources can
complement the work of health providers
in responding to gender-based violence and
how these groups can work together most
effectively to transform community norms
and attitudes. ⌒

Chapter Seven

Beyond the Clinic: Violence Prevention
with Other Community Partners

One of the most important lessons that health providers have learned, as they take on gender-based violence in their daily practice, is that no one profession or group can eliminate violence working on its own. Although national policies, laws, and programs are necessary to create a supportive environment for change, the real work of violence prevention takes place in the communities themselves. In many different geographical settings visited by the review team, the health care providers who reported having the most positive experiences in addressing GBV attributed much of their success to close coordination with other local leaders, government institutions, and NGOs based in their own communities.

The principal community-based activities carried out as part of the PAHO project were the following:

* training health leaders and promoters;
* strengthening local networks for coordinating violence prevention efforts;
* public education, within and outside the clinical setting;
* reflection groups with men; and
* support groups for women survivors of violence.

This chapter presents the achievements and constraints of the various PAHO GBV programs and initiatives from the perspective of community participants and clients. In order to gain the perspective of stakeholders outside the health sector, the assessment team met with community health leaders and midwives, women's groups, and other organizations participating in both local and national commissions for violence prevention. Participatory techniques such as the use of timelines and Venn diagrams were used to encourage participants to talk candidly about the community forces that have helped or hindered violence prevention efforts. These techniques and the information they yielded will be described in this chapter.

COMMUNITY HEALTH PROMOTERS
Sensitizing community leaders (traditional birth attendants, legal advocates, health promoters, etc.) about GBV was considered an important strategy for engaging community members in violence prevention in all countries. The intensity of training and awareness-building initiatives varied among the countries, as well as the specific activities performed by community promoters. In some communities the promoters only referred cases to the police or health centers, whereas in other settings they had been trained to offer crisis intervention and legal counseling and even to accompany women

through the legal process. The community volunteers provide an important link between health services and the communities. In most cases health promoters also carry out educational activities on violence prevention and provide women with information about their legal rights and other available community services.

In the Justo Rufino Barrios Clinic in Guatemala City, health promoters perform short theatrical skits in the waiting rooms as a way of introducing the topic of violence and encouraging patients to talk to their providers if they need help. Because health leaders, and particularly traditional birth attendants, are well-respected in their communities, they are particularly well-positioned to be able to influence views and behavior.

LESSONS LEARNED
Community health leaders have a crucial role to play in violence prevention, through the promotion of nonviolent relationships, and by informing the community and women in particular about their legal and social rights and providing information and appropriate referrals to abused women. In addition to providing appropriate training, health providers should work together with community health leaders to agree upon the roles and responsibilities of all actors. Providers should also meet regularly with community volunteers to ensure that they are receiving sufficient support in their work.

"I helped a woman who felt smaller than a cock-
roach because her husband wanted to take away
her house and the children. I took her to the
health center, and after she talked to them her
burden was lighter."
—Community health worker, El Salvador

The training sessions for community promoters commonly address a broad range
of issues, such as different types of violence
and their impact on the health of women
and children, and include a discussion of
gender roles and how gender-based discrimination encourages violence. The participants also gain a greater understanding
of how the legal system works and what
options are available to victims of violence
in their own communities.

In many health centers that have programs
for community health promotion, the GBV
training is carried out as part of a larger,
more comprehensive training that includes
aspects of reproductive and child health,
environmental sanitation, and other basic
health topics. In some settings, however,
community women were invited to workshops on violence prevention and became
so motivated by the training sessions that
they started their own violence programs.
For example, a group of traditional birth
attendants in the town of Santa Lucía,
Guatemala, created their own violence prevention organization and obtained support
from the local mayor's office as well as the
health center to provide counseling for
abused women. After the creation of the
Luciana Women's Group, many women felt
for the first time that there was someone
they could turn to with their problems. After
the group members had received additional
training through the PAHO project, health
personnel would refer women to them, and
the group even set up an office within the
health center itself and the members took

turns staffing the service. One of the
strengths of this approach was that women
felt more comfortable talking to someone
with a background similar to their own:

". . . Women felt supported by the women's
office that was in the mayor's office, and they
used to say to their husband, 'if you hit me
I'll take you to the office....'"
—Traditional birth attendant, Santa Lucía,
Guatemala

". . . Women, when they begin to talk about their
situation of violence, want someone to tell them
what to do, because they feel disoriented, with
very low self-esteem, and they need economic help."
—Traditional birth attendant, Santa Lucía,
Guatemala

Another group of Mayan women from the
town of Totonicapán in Guatemala, feeling
that the government offices would be unable
to respond adequately to the needs of indigenous women, created their own center for
abused women with international support.

". . . In the indigenous communities of
Guatemala, even though women are informed
about the laws, it is not enough, because the
community leaders, mostly men, have a lot of
influence on women's decisions, and their view
is that violence is 'normal' among couples. . . . "
—Educator from Cobán, Guatemala

"Women feel much better when they are accompanied to the courts and the police station by
the project's legal promoters because they feel
that they are not alone and that they are being
listened to. . . ."
—Mayan midwife from Totonicapán, Guatemala

In other communities, particularly in
El Salvador and Nicaragua, services for
abused women offered by local women's
groups already existed when the PAHO

project started, although in most cases there was previously little coordination between these groups and local health services. In these cases, the goal of the PAHO project was to encourage health providers to reach out to the groups already working on violence, to learn from them, and to begin to coordinate with them in prevention activities and care for the survivors. Health providers in communities where work on violence was already ongoing found that the existence of these resources made it much easier for their own programs to take hold.

COMMUNITY-BASED NETWORKS

PAHO's integrated approach for addressing GBV has placed great emphasis on the development of community-based networks for violence prevention. The Critical Path study found that improving coordination between institutions that deal with GBV was an essential step to improving care for survivors, who, in most cases, were forced to maneuver their way through enormously complicated and duplicative procedures in each institution, which, as this book has shown, caused many women to become discouraged and eventually abandon their search for help.

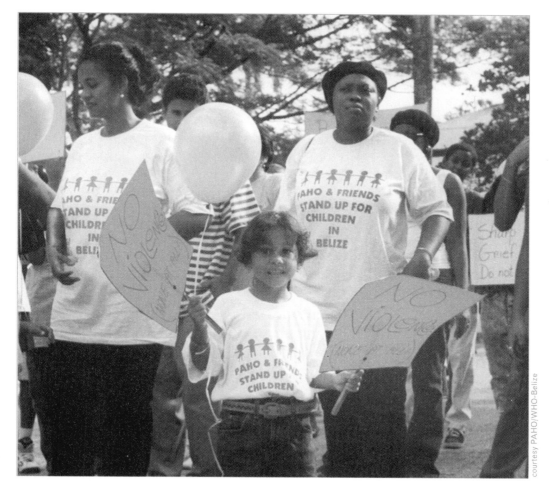

Community demonstration against violence in Belize

Community-based networks have two major goals—to provide a comprehensive range of services that effectively meets the needs of survivors of violence, which can be achieved by improving communication and coordination between groups working on GBV; and secondly, to raise public awareness and transform community attitudes that encourage and/or tolerate violence.

When the PAHO GBV project first began, there was a wide disparity between the countries with regard to the levels of GBV interest and awareness among local institutions. In some countries, such as Nicaragua, violence prevention networks had already been operating for many years, and the main challenge was motivating health personnel to participate in them. In other cases, health workers, with the help of the PAHO project, took the initiative to bring community groups and institutions together for the first time. To date, there is still a great deal of dissimilarity among the countries with regard to how highly developed the networks are. In Guatemala, for example, where there is very little tradition of coordination between state institutions and civil society, community leaders noted that it has been a struggle to maintain ongoing coordination among the different governmental actors, such as the police, judges, and the health sector, and even more difficult to coordinate actions with women's groups. Providers and women's activists reported that periodical efforts were made to increase coordination, but that these tended to dissipate fairly quickly. In the town of Comayagua, Honduras, coordination between the Family Counseling Center and other institutions dealing with violence (the Human Rights Commission, police, child welfare bureau, etc.) was very strong. However, network members reported that they did not meet regularly as a group, or plan activities jointly, but rather settled

specific issues on an ad hoc basis as the need arose.

In order to understand how community members—both clients and the service providers themselves—view the different types of support available to survivors of violence, a participatory technique called "Who Helps Rosita," based on the use of Venn diagrams, was carried out in the various project communites visited (see Figures 7-1., 7-2., and 7-3.). This exercise compares the relative support provided by state institutions, community services, and individuals. Different sized and colored circles were used to represent these and other groups who could potentially help Rosita, who, as we saw in Chapter Six's introductory section, is a mother of two children and lives with her abusive husband. The darker colored circles indicated government institutions, and the lighter ones represented nongovernmental groups, such as women's organizations, church groups, friends, relatives, and neighbors. The participants were asked to assess each of the groups according to how helpful they found them to be (represented by the size of the circle—the larger the circle, the more helpful), and how responsive they were (the closer the circles' proximity to Rosita, the more responsive they were considered to be to her needs).

There was a clear relationship between the strength of local networks and the women's perceptions of the number and types of institutions that they could turn to for help. In two sessions with Guatemalan activists—one with community health leaders in a peri-urban neighborhood of Guatemala City and another with indigenous women activists from the rural town of Totonicapán—the participants' views of state institutions were quite similar, despite the differences between the two settings (Figures 7-1. and 7-2.). In both cases, participants considered church groups and family networks to be the most important sources of support for abused women. At the same time, the health center—and specifically the GBV personnel—were considered to be the only government-run services that were responsive to women. In general, all other institutions that might be expected to help abused women, such as the police, the courts, forensic doctors, etc., were categorized as either unavailable or not helpful.

Not surprisingly, in both settings, health providers acknowledged that it had been very difficult to build institutional networks for the coordination of GBV work, since the other institutions seemed unwilling to commit the time and effort needed to create and sustain them.

A very different situation was found in the rural town of Apopa, in El Salvador, where the director of the health center brought together more than 20 members of the local violence prevention commission, including the town's mayor, police chief, NGO representatives, and district health officials, to discuss its work with the review team. Although participants acknowledged that the commission had, at best, functioned only on an intermittent basis, its formation had clearly generated a higher level of enthusiasm and concern around the issue. Interestingly, this was reflected in the results of a focus group discussion with women clients of the Chintúc Health Center in Apopa. These women were able to name several government institutions, as well as NGOs and women's groups, who could assist abused women (Figure 7-3.). Many of them had personally been helped or else knew someone who had been helped by the police or the local courts. They told many stories in which the police had been sup-

portive of women living in violent situations even when family members and neighbors had not offered them help.

"When the family took his side, the police told them to stay out of it, and they didn't let his mother go to the station with him."
—Health promoter, Apopa, El Salvador

WHAT MAKES A COMMUNITY NETWORK SUCCESSFUL?

Of the four countries visited during the review, Nicaragua has the longest and richest experience with community networks for violence prevention. Even in the towns where efforts to address GBV in the health center were just getting underway, they benefited enormously from the already-established tradition of strong community participation and coordination.

Nicaragua's experience is unique in several respects. To begin with, there has been an

---

LESSONS LEARNED
The establishment of community networks can greatly help in coordinating services for victims of violence and in developing joint programs for violence prevention. In all of the countries reviewed, women's organizations and related groups have played a pivotal role in consolidating the networks. In addition, different sectors have played key roles in specific countries: for example, the National Police Force, through the Women and Children's Police Stations, have been the driving force for coordination in Nicaragua, whereas in Belize, Costa Rica, and Panama, the health sector has played a prominent role.

FIGURE 7-1. WHO HELPS ROSITA?

Opinions of Mayan women from Totonicapán towards institutions and groups working with gender-based violence in Guatemala, using Venn diagrams. Darker circles indicate government institutions, and the lighter ones represent nongovernmental groups, such as women's organizations, church groups, friends, neighbors, and relatives. The more helpful the group the larger the circle and the closer its proximity to Rosita. Positive and negative signs (+/-) placed together indicate that the experience with this group could be either positive or negative, depending on the particular situation.

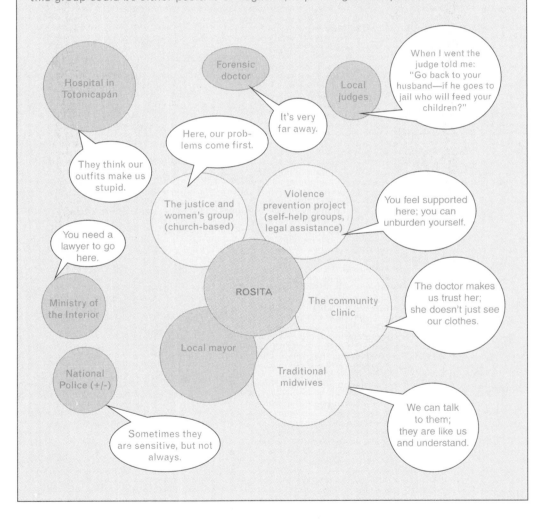

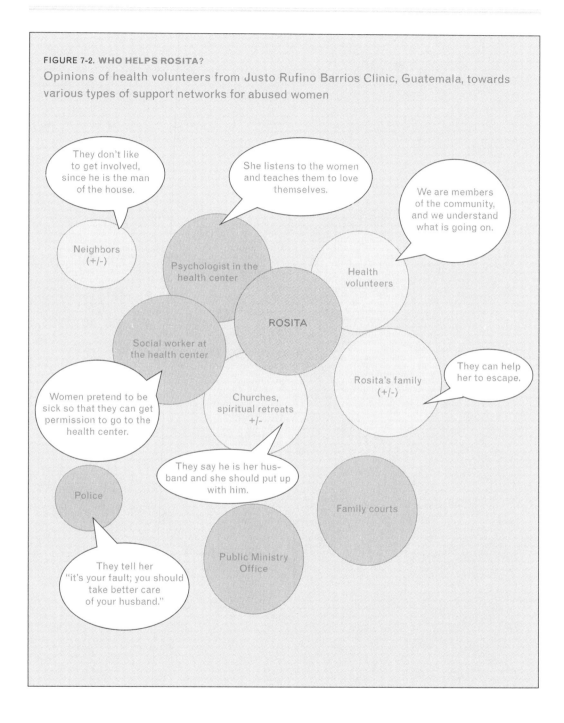

FIGURE 7-2. WHO HELPS ROSITA?

Opinions of health volunteers from Justo Rufino Barrios Clinic, Guatemala, towards various types of support networks for abused women

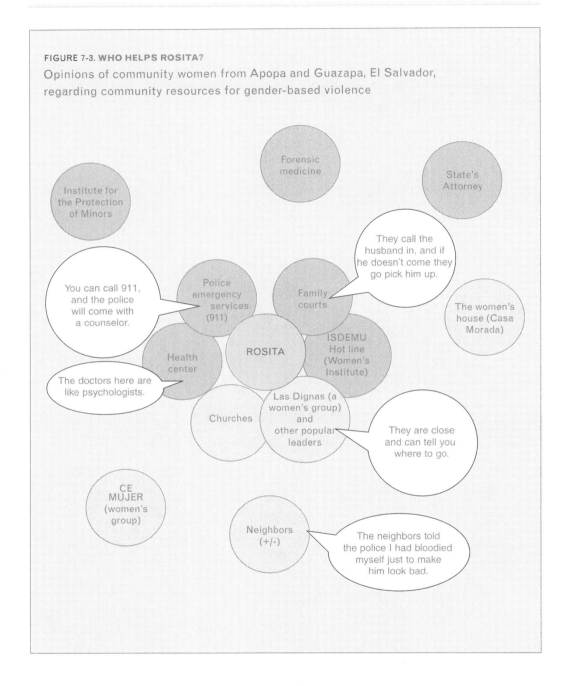

FIGURE 7-3. WHO HELPS ROSITA?
Opinions of community women from Apopa and Guazapa, El Salvador, regarding community resources for gender-based violence

extensive organized movement of women's organizations working with GBV for more than 10 years. Over 100 organizations throughout the country participate in the National Network of Women against Violence, which also has regional networks in most of the major cities and towns. The Network carries out yearly national awareness campaigns; it drafted and successfully lobbied for the passage in 1997 of the Family Violence Law; and network members play an active ongoing role in the development and monitoring of the Women and Children's Police Stations. It also has a research and health commission, which, in 1995, together with the Medical School of UNAN-León, performed the first population-based study on the prevalence of domestic violence in Central America (Ellsberg et al. 2000). The group also has produced educational materials on GBV, including a training manual for health workers used widely throughout the country (Red de Mujeres contra la Violencia 1999). In several districts, members of the local violence networks have helped to train health workers in GBV.

Without a doubt, a major force that has shaped work on GBV in Nicaragua is the creation of the 17 Women and Children's Police Stations (*Comisarías*) that currently function in all the major cities throughout the country. The stations are staffed by trained women police officers and social workers and have been financed primarily through international support. In addition to receiving and investigating complaints of violence, the police stations work together with local NGOs to provide rehabilitation services and public education on violence. Whenever a *Comisaría* is set up, local networks are established to provide technical support and oversight for its work. Network members also receive training and other

resources for prevention activities and services that have contributed greatly to the strength of the *Comisarías* as well as to the community networks.

In Nicaragua, the review team met with the local violence prevention networks in Chinandega, in the country's northwestern corner; Bluefields, on the Atlantic Coast; and Estelí, a town in the country's northern area.

In addition to being the first pilot site for the PAHO project, Estelí was one of the first cities to establish a Women and Children's Police Station. There are five different nongovernmental centers in the town that provide psychological, legal, and/or medical services for survivors of violence, including *Acción Ya*, Nicaragua's first shelter for abused women. In addition to these centers, a Commision for Violence Prevention has been created that includes the local and district judges, the district attorney, and representatives of the Ministries of Health, Education, and the Family. Using an exercise called "The Road Traveled," members of the network described the most important moments in their history and placed these in chronological order along a timeline, with positive events on the top half of the line and factors that negatively influenced the process on the bottom (Figure 7-4.).

In Estelí the process began in 1995 with the establishment of the Women and Children's Police Station. According to the group, the achievements that most contributed to the consolidation of its work were:

→ carrying out joint training workshops for all members of the network (police, judges, and youth groups);

→ travel exchanges with other countries to learn from their experiences (for example,

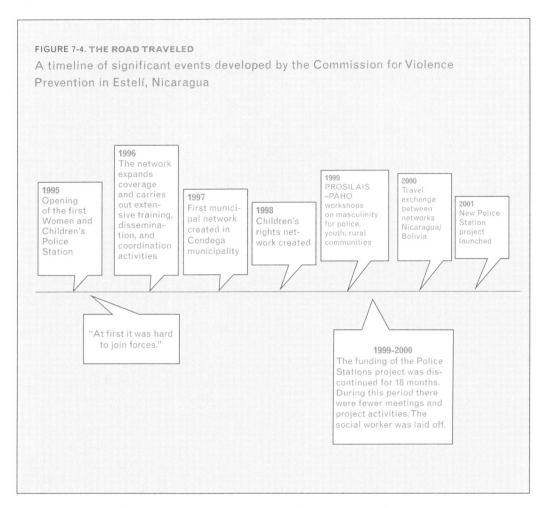

FIGURE 7-4. **THE ROAD TRAVELED**

A timeline of significant events developed by the Commission for Violence Prevention in Estelí, Nicaragua

a PAHO-supported exchange between the Estelí network and a town in Bolivia);

➔ the creation of municipal networks in the smaller towns surrounding Estelí, such as Condega, which increased the scope of the GBV work considerably;

➔ setting up a national training program in Esteli, where professionals from other regions can learn from the experiences of all of the centers participating in the program; and

➔ establishing a local initiative in which area groups contributed time and resources to keep the Women and Children's Police

Station running during a period when international funding had been discontinued.

By developing joint plans for training and public awareness activities, the Estelí network was able to optimize scarce funding and to leverage funding from other sources, such as the PROSILAIS health reform project funded by the Swedish Government, which financed the study tours of health professionals from other regions in the country to Estelí.

Another example of effective leveraging of resources is the newly formed violence prevention commission in Bluefields. The Ministry of Health representatives have played a key role in strengthening the commission's work by sharing resources with other members to carry out sensitivity training on GBV to professionals working in other sectors that have a strong influence on community attitudes, such as teachers, judges, and religious leaders. After participating in sensitivity workshops, teachers are asked to sign a pledge listing the outreach activities they plan to carry out together with their students and colleagues.

While not visited by the review team, the indigenous town of El Alto in Bolivia also offers another interesting example of the potential of well-integrated community violence prevention networks to score impressive gains in mobilizing resources and raising public awareness around the issue of violence (Box 7-1.).

INCORPORATING MEN IN CHANGING THE CULTURE OF VIOLENCE

In most countries that the review team visited, both providers and clients underscored the importance of encouraging the participation of men in all violence prevention activities, pointing out that it is not possible to eliminate violence against women if the attitudes and behavior of violent men are not changed as a central part of this process.

Providers noted that abused women often request help for their husbands—someone to provide the men with guidance and counseling to help motivate them to change. These women do not necessarily want to end their relationships; what they want is for the violence to end. This is one of the reasons why out-of-court arrangements incorporating these types of services are requested more frequently than criminal prosecution.

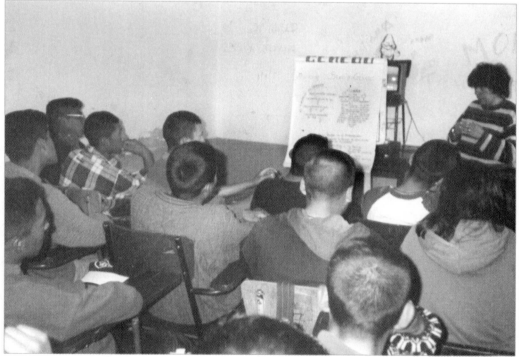

courtesy PAHO/WHO-Bolivia

New recruits in the Bolivian armed forces are instructed in GBV sensitization as part of their basic military training.

BOX 7-1. THE EXPERIENCE OF BOLIVIA:
THE NETWORK FOR THE PREVENTION AND CARE OF FAMILY VIOLENCE

In September 1998, in the city of El Alto, Bolivia, a group of governmental, nongovernmental, and community organizations formed the Network for the Prevention and Care
of Family Violence. Together they developed a work plan and set up committees for
implementing the plan and for mobilizing technical and financial resources among the
member organizations.

Since its beginning, the Network has been successful in coordinating the work of a
wide variety of city government entities, such as the Office of Gender Affairs, the
Office of Social Administration, the health center, the public defender's office, the
police unit responding to family-related and emergency situations, the local team of
Doctors without Borders, and a confederation of more than 100 grassroots organizations.

With their shared agenda these members worked together to achieve the following:
- In 2001, members registered 15,371 cases of violence out of a total population of
  98,670 women.
- The health center recorded 297 cases of family violence, of which 36% were referred
  to the police and/or other legal authorities. Before there was no reporting of this type.

**DEMAND FOR LEGAL SERVICES FOR DOMESTIC VIOLENCE
EL ALTO, BOLIVIA, 1997-2001**

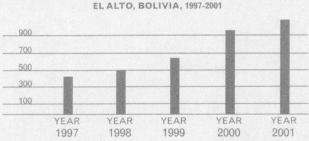

courtesy Gregoria Apaza Center for the Promotion of Women

The lessons learned are:

- Effective systems for collecting and analyzing information on gender-based violence
  are critical for determining the problem's scope; for raising awareness among service
  providers, particularly from the health sector; and for influencing political decision-
  making at the local level.
- Partnerships among governmental, nongovernmental, and local organizations that
  are built on sustained commitment and incorporate each member's expertise are
  essential for the delivery of well-integrated and high-quality services.
- The community's ethnic identity, of predominately Aymara origins, must be recognized and incorporated in the targeting of interventions and in the promotion of rights
  and equity.

Dora Caballero, PAHO/WHO-Bolivia

In Canada, Europe, and the United States, there are many treatment programs for abusers that include a variety of theoretical and programmatic approaches. Most programs have a duration of 8–12 weeks. The participants are sent to the programs as an alternative sentence by the courts. Few evaluations have been conducted to measure the effectiveness of this strategy. Attendance data, however, indicate that approximately half of the men drop out before completing the program. Of those that do finish, approximately half of them stop using physical violence, at least for some period of time. However, in many cases they continue to display other forms of violent and/or controlling behavior. One key for success is the participant's motivation. Not surprisingly, men who participate voluntarily (for example, because they don't want to lose their family and/or end their relationship or because they feel true remorse about their actions) are more likely to change than those who participate in a program they basically feel is punitive in its intent (Edleson 1995).

In Honduras and Panama, family violence laws require the health sector to provide treatment for offenders, and the courts may use attendance to an abusers' treatment program as an alternative sentence. In Honduras, the review team visited a program for male abusers and interviewed the wives of some of the participants who attended therapy sessions at the Family Counseling Center (see Box 7-2.). It appeared that some men did use the opportunity to reflect on their behavior, while many others were merely "counting down the hours" until their sentence was completed, without ever assuming any real responsibility for their actions. Some of the wives described positive changes in their husbands' behavior and actions as a result of the program, although one woman who had

lost consciousness more than once due to the brutality of her husband's assaults confessed: "I still feel afraid of him."

During its assessment, the review team found several areas of potential concern regarding the laws requiring the health system to treat offenders:

→ No additional resources are allocated for these services; therefore, there is the risk of diverting funds that would otherwise be available for treating violence victims.

→ The Honduran law establishes a kind of symmetry between male offenders and female survivors. Women are also obliged to attend counseling sessions, with the goal of "increasing their self-esteem." Just as the offenders, they can be punished with mandatory community service if they fail to attend. A psychologist at the Colonia Kennedy Family Counseling Center noted that one woman who had been assaulted by her husband was now in danger of losing her job because of the mandatory therapy sessions and that she had been unable to obtain a deferral from the judge. Although the intention of the measure is positive, obligating the victim of a crime to receive treatment against her will violates the most important principle of care for survivors; that is, to strengthen a sense of personal autonomy. Moreover, it was evident in discussions with offenders that they viewed this measure as an "official" acknowledgment that men and women are equally responsible for the violence.

→ There is no consensus among mental health professionals in these two countries (or elsewhere in the project countries studied) regarding the theoretical and methodological guidelines for treating male offenders. Therefore, the lack of norms

BOX 7-2. "YOU NEVER EXPECT YOUR WIFE TO DO THIS TO YOU. . . ."
EXPERIENCES FROM A MEN'S GROUP IN HONDURAS

The review team interviewed 30 men in an offenders' group run by the Family Counseling Center of Colonia Kennedy, Tegucigalpa. All of these men attend a weekly two-hour session for eight weeks by order by the courts. They acknowledged that they would not have participated if they had not been required to do so. Most felt themselves to be victims of the criminal justice system. Only one man admitted to ever having hit his wife. Another man explained that he had filed charges against his wife under the family violence law, "because she nagged me too much," and the judge required him to attend the groups instead.

"The judge here is biased against us. Even if the wife wants to find a solution the judge does not help settle things. She treats men badly; then if the wife is listening, it gives her ideas."

"When I was in front of the judge, my wife became bold and tough."

In terms of the negative attention by the judge toward male aggressors, the men suggested that having a male judge for the men would be a fairer approach, "as they understand one another better," and having a female judge for the women.

A few men acknowledged some benefits from attending the groups, despite the unpleasantness of being obligated to attend.

"You never expect your wife to do this to you; even so, I have learned something here, and my behavior will be different in the future. You realize that not everything you do is right; for example, thinking that a wife is her husband's property."

"The first time you attend, it's hard to talk. Here, everyone can tell their own version of things. You feel relieved when you tell the truth. That helps; it's one less burden, and you stop believing that you know everything and you're a good person."

"I felt some hatred towards women before this [due to previous abuse by his mother]. Then, thank God, my wife turned me in [to the police], and now my life is different; I've left that burden behind."

and trained personnel for the treatment of offenders in these cases may only further jeopardize the women's safety.

→ There is little capacity for case follow-up to determine the effectiveness of the programs.

A Nicaraguan group, the Association of Men against Violence, has developed an innovative proposal to work with "men who have problems with power and control in their intimate relationships." This group explicitly addresses the problem of power and control because it considers male violence to be merely one characteristic of relationships based on the subordination of one partner by another. With this approach the group aims to avoid the "trap" that

LESSONS LEARNED

Abusers' treatment groups should not be confused with men's reflection groups. The purpose of the reflection groups is to encourage men (either community members or health workers) to challenge prevailing cultural views on masculinity and to become more sensitive to gender-equitable norms. Men's groups can be an effective way to involve both adults and young men in violence prevention activities.

In contrast, most health services are not equipped to manage abusers' treatment groups, particularly when the courts mandate attendance as an alternative sentence. These programs require a different methodology and trained personnel, and if poorly managed, can put women at even greater risk. Ideally, the criminal justice system or professionals outside the public health system should manage these groups.

some programs fall into by focusing exclusively on eliminating physical violence, while ignoring other more subtle forms of domination. This program targets male volunteers who have not already been prosecuted or sentenced for assault; i.e., those men who presumably are somewhat more likely to accept messages of reciprocity than men who have already entered into the justice system.

The Nicaraguan proposal establishes a clear difference between men's reflection groups and abusers' groups; they feel that different methods are warranted in each case. In some of the other Central American experiences, the distinctions between the two types of groups appear to be more blurred.

The main purpose of the Nicaraguan abusers' groups is to enhance "the security of women and children. [The program's goal] is to treat men in order to first benefit women and children, and then men." As one member of the Association noted,

"In the abusers' groups there is no agreement to keep the discussions confidential. This means we are able to verify whether men have changed their attitudes and behavior by checking with their partners. Men who participate in the group have to agree to this rule."

CHANGING COMMUNITY NORMS ON VIOLENCE

As discussed in Chapter One of this book, one of the major findings of international research on the causes of GBV is that, although individual risk factors, such as witnessing violence as a child, poverty, or use of alcohol, may increase a specific individual's likelihood to use violence, cultural norms play a large role in overall levels of violence in a community. In many parts of the world, it is considered both a right and even an obligation for men to physically chastise their wives in the face of perceived transgressions. A man's honor often depends on his ability to control his wife's behavior. In a study performed by the Nicaraguan Network of Women against Violence, a rural man explained how to beat his wife without leaving visible scars that might get him in trouble with the police:

"You have to know just how to give it to a woman. Women should be hit where it doesn't show, and preferably on the bottom with a belt or using the flat end of a machete. . . . This isn't serious because it can't be seen; but if I hit her in the eye, that's a problem. . . ."
—Ellsberg, Liljestrand, and Winkvist 1997

Community-based educational activities can increase women's knowledge of legal and social rights and empower them to seek help for abuse. They can also challenge the underlying beliefs that justify women's subordination and the use of violence for settling conflicts. Promoting nonviolent and equitable relationships between men and women is the key to preventing future violence.

Over the last 10 years, numerous groups in Nicaragua have carried out national campaigns against violence. The Nicaraguan Network of Women against Violence carries out a yearly campaign that combines mass media messages on popular television and radio shows with local activities, petitions, and buttons with popular slogans (Box 7-3.).

A Nicaraguan NGO, the *Puntos de Encuentro* Foundation, has also carried out national media campaigns targeting different groups, such as one encouraging men to be more equitable in their relationships and to find new ways to resolve conflicts (Figure 7-6.).

A Demographic and Health survey performed in 1998 found that nearly half of all Nicaraguan women had seen or heard at

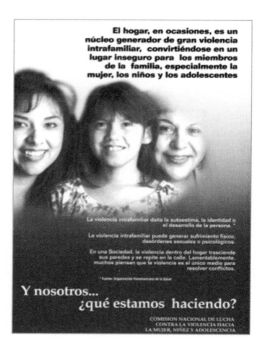

FIGURE 7-5. CAMPAIGN BY THE NICARAGUAN COMMISSION ON VIOLENCE AGAINST WOMEN noting that the home can become the nucleus for violence against women, adolescents, and children

least one of the messages, and that of these, almost half of the women could repeat at least one of them (Rosales et al. 1999).

Puntos de Encuentro also produces a television program called *Sexto sentido* (Sixth Sense) targeting adolescents of both sexes. The show, which has received top ratings among its youthful viewers, addresses a variety of issues, such as sexuality, generational conflicts, gender equity, and violence against women and children. In an evaluation of the program, a young woman said:

". . . After watching *Sexto sentido* I knew what to do when a friend told me that she had been sexually abused by someone in her family. I followed the same steps as the girl in the show, and I gave her the telephone numbers they show so that she could talk to someone who was better informed."
—*Puntos de Encuentro* 2002

be easily hidden and provide basic information about the domestic violence law, how to prepare a safety plan, and where to go for help.

Many of the centers visited by the review team had posters displayed about violence and/or distributed brochures to their clients about violence, but few of these had been developed specifically for health care settings. Instead, most had been produced by local women's groups or international human rights organizations. Several health workers suggested that ministries of health and PAHO should develop a regionwide public awareness campaign specifically addressing GBV as a health problem and encouraging women to talk to their providers about violence. "We need to create a comfortable environment in the health center, with messages saying that we care about violence," observed a nurse in Bluefields, Nicaragua. One of the women interviewed in El Salvador explained that the main reason she went to the health center

Health centers can also provide an ideal setting for spreading messages about violence. In the United States, many health professionals prominently display posters or wear buttons that tell clients "You can talk to me about violence" (Heise, Ellsberg, and Gottemoeller 1999). In Peru, the Ministry of Health, in conjunction with the Flora Tristán Center and PAHO, developed small table tents to be placed on providers' desks (Figure 7-7.). The side facing clients notes: "No one has the right to mistreat you. If you suffer violence in your home, your health is being seriously affected. Talk to us about it." The reverse side reminds providers to take the opportunity to talk about violence with their clients. The Nicaraguan Network of Women against Violence produced small cards for providers to give their clients with the title, "If you are living with violence, there are ways out." The cards are small enough to

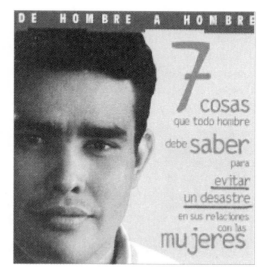

FIGURE 7-6. "SEVEN THINGS EVERY MAN
SHOULD KNOW TO AVOID A DISASTER IN
HIS RELATIONSHIPS WITH WOMEN,"
an anti-violence campaign targeting men
carried out by the *Puntos de Encuentro*
Foundation, Nicaragua

with her problems was that she had seen a handwritten sign on the wall that said "We help victims of domestic violence here."

SUPPORT GROUPS FOR SURVIVORS

Support groups are effective and low-cost techniques for helping survivors overcome their experiences of violence. In the Americas, there are several organizations, for example, CEFEMINA (*Centro Feminista de Información y Acción*) in Costa Rica and the Flora Tristán Center in Peru, with extensive experience in organizing self-help or support groups for violence survivors.

One of the main advantages of support groups is that they enable centers to respond to many more individuals than would be possible with individual psychological care. Additionally, the group facilitator does not have to be a mental health professional, although special training is necessary. Another advantage is that women are given the opportunity to help each other; to realize that they are not the only ones that suffer from violence; to develop common ties; and in some cases, to even take collective action. These are all important factors in helping women sustain their resolve to overcome violence.

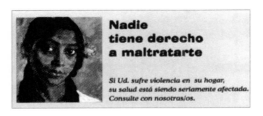

FIGURE 7-7. TABLE TENT USED IN PERU to encourage women to discuss violence with health providers. The text says: "No one has the right to mistreat you. If you suffer violence in your home, your health is being seriously affected. Talk to us about it."

PAHO has promoted the development of support groups through staff training and distribution of educational materials. In each project country, there has been at least one attempt to create an ongoing program of support groups. One important aspect of this process observed by the review team was that the success of support groups did not appear to depend on the level of specialized personnel; there were successful groups in one health post managed by an auxiliary nurse, while some centers equipped with specialized mental health teams assured the team that it would be impossible to establish groups of this type in their communities. The main difficulties cited by health providers included:

"In rural communities everyone knows one another, and they don't want to expose their personal lives to others because of embarrassment or fear of retaliation by their husbands."
—Comayagua, Honduras

"We have no specialized personnel to facilitate the groups."
—Chinandega, Nicaragua

"We tried to create a group but the women did not want to attend; they are not interested."
—Santa Lucía, Guatemala

In general, it appears that the success or failure of support groups has much more to do with the motivation and skill of the individual health workers than with the characteristics of a particular community or the professional training of facilitators. In most project countries one or two workshops had been held to train facilitators, but these professionals have received little additional training or follow-up support. The lack of experience of facilitators, coupled with the fear of failure, are a significant barrier for the success of the support groups. As one psychologist from Guatemala observed:

BOX 7-4. IMPORTANT QUALITIES FOR FACILITATORS OF SUPPORT GROUPS

-Training in gender and violence
-Training in the dynamics of abuse, different types of abuse, and their consequences
-Familiarity with strategies for empowerment and recuperation
-Training in ethical norms for working with violence against women and knowledge of existing laws

From: Claramunt 1999

BOX 7-5. WHAT WE HAVE LEARNED IN SUPPORT GROUPS

-To be independent
-To value ourselves
-To be more responsible with our children
-To make responsible decisions for ourselves
-To recognize our qualities
-Not to be violent
-To develop self-esteem
-To put our abilities into practice
-To say, "I am competent, I can do it"
-To empower ourselves
-To have our rights respected and not be abused
-To love ourselves
-To forgive
-To liberate ourselves
-To respect
-To love
-To have solidarity within the group

Statements from support group, Barrio Lourdes, El Salvador

". . . It is important not to scold the women . . . . In order to facilitate a support group you need to be trained and learn to deal with your own experiences of violence. . . ."

Nevertheless, in the sites where support groups continue to operate, the health personnel as well as the participants are convinced that they are an excellent technique for helping survivors of violence.

The polyclinic of Barrio Lourdes in El Salvador operates a comprehensive program with several support groups for survivors of violence, including one for elderly women. What is noteworthy about this experience is that a physical therapist and special education therapist facilitate the groups, although the center has several psychologists on staff. The facilitators were chosen not for their professional background but because of their interest in and commitment to the topic and their ability to develop trust with their clients.

A Guatemalan psychologist found group support to be more beneficial to women than individual counseling because of the bonds that are created among the participants:

"The solidarity of the women is admirable. They give each other ideas for moving forward. Group sessions produce better results. After a few sessions they start asking each other, 'Have you tried such-and-such?' Personally, seeing how the women talk to each other with such wisdom has helped me to understand the problem better. . . .

"The important thing is that the groups are anonymous; not everyone knows everyone else. You don't have to be Superman to facilitate a group; instead [just] begin with patience, and don't scold them. . . . The main ground rule of the group is that 'We are not here to gossip, but to work on our problems.'"

> ## LESSONS LEARNED
> Support groups can be a very effective technique for helping violence survivors.
>
> Nevertheless, health personnel do need training and ongoing support to be effective facilitators.

An auxiliary nurse from Guazapa, El Salvador, described her experience this way:

"It took a lot of work to create this group. After receiving individual care, each woman is invited to join. We started with 12 women, then the number decreased. We now have 6 women that meet every 15 days. I have had to fight with my boss to have the time to care for them. I have also taught them handicrafts, which they have enjoyed."

The indigenous promoters from Totonicapán, Guatemala, also noted that offering to teach the women practical skills provided additional incentive for their participation:

". . . The groups are working well, but our strategy is to include classes on cooking and traditional medicine so that more women will come and their husbands won't be suspicious about their participation. . . ."

The following comments of women who have participated in support groups provide a moving testimony to the importance of the groups. The main comment heard over and over from survivors who had come into contact with caring health providers, either in groups or in individual sessions, was how important it was for them to feel that someone cared and was willing to listen, and then could give them information and encouragement that bolstered their sense of self-worth and knowledge about their rights.

"I used to think that death was the only way out. I wanted to die but I couldn't kill myself because of my children. . . . I thought it was my fault that he hit me. Here, I've learned that it's not so . . . my self-esteem was very low, [but] here they teach us to love ourselves. . . ."
—Colonia Kennedy, Honduras

"I used to be very shy. I was enslaved in the house. . . . Now, thanks to the group, I feel liberated."
—Comayagua, Honduras

"What helped me was to realize that I wasn't alone. There are many of us who feel trapped and silenced inside ourselves. Learning about laws and communicating among ourselves were also very important to help us break our silence."
—Colonia Kennedy, Honduras

EXPANDING THE CIRCLE

The narratives presented in Section II of this book have been selected to help the reader come away with a greater appreciation for and understanding of what the review team considers to be the single most all-encompassing lesson learned from the PAHO project evaluation: that individuals and institutions, working together in an integrated approach, can harness enormous power to transform not only their own

---

> **BOX 7-5. WHAT ADVICE WOULD YOU GIVE WOMEN WHO ARE LIVING WITH VIOLENCE?**
>
> - Love your children
> - Go to the health center to be listened to
> - You need to want a change
> - You matter and are important
> - Be independent
> - Know your rights
>
> _____
> *Statements by women from*
> *Barrios Lourdes support group in El Salvador*

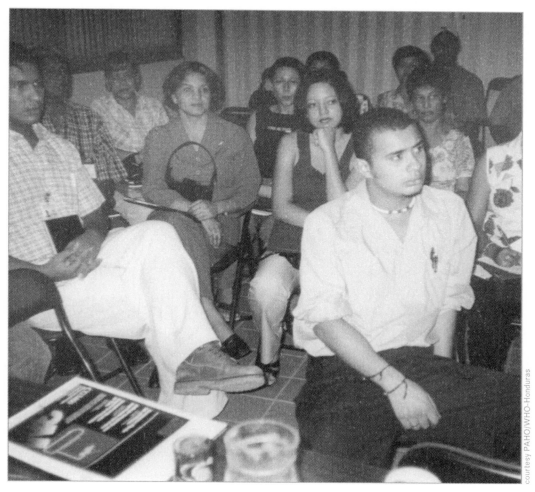

courtesy PAHO/WHO-Honduras

Incorporating men in open discussions on GBV, such as this one in Honduras, is an effective strategy that can be used by community groups to promote the idea that violence prevention and mutual respect are everyone's responsibility.

thoughts, feelings, and actions, but also those of the communities where they live. While a central theme of this book has been the importance of the health sector taking a lead role in galvanizing this process, the review team also found abundant evidence of the need for true cooperation and binding partnerships with other key sectors to consolidate and institutionalize the initiatives currently underway. If this goal is achieved, the circle can be widened within communities and the dynamic extended to new ones.

In Chapter Eight, these stories and lessons will be placed and explored within a larger context: that of other communities around the world. The collective experiences can provide both a theoretical and practical blueprint for dedicated individuals and groups, wherever they may be, who wish to embark on a similar journey and who seek solidarity, inspiration, and guidance in their own efforts to rid our societies of violence and create a new international culture of true equality between women and men. ☞

Chapter Eight

Global Implications:
The PAHO Approach to Gender-Based Violence

WOMEN ARE WAITING FOR THE WORLD TO RESPOND

The women in the pages of this book who described lives filled with physical and emotional abuse are not unique. In fact, their suffering is mirrored back to us in every language and from every corner of the world. In the words of Kofi Annan, Secretary General of the United Nations, violence against women is "the most pervasive human rights violation, respecting no distinction of geography, culture, or wealth" (U.N. Secretary General SG/SM/6334). What has changed is that in the last few years there has been a growing awareness and acceptance that the problem exists, and with it, a more palpable commitment to identifying and addressing its roots.

GBV has long been of concern to both the World Health Organization (WHO) and PAHO. Both have given the issue high priority in their work with national governments and grassroots advocacy at the community level. Both are aware of the opportunities available for public health to play a central role in turning the tide against violence and of the responsibilities the health sector can and must assume in this pivotal role.

In 1995, WHO, in its position paper presented at the Fourth World Conference on Women in Beijing, identified violence against women as a priority issue for women's health (WHO 1995). Meanwhile, PAHO's Women, Health, and Development Program had already started work in this area, following the passage in 1993 of a resolution urging PAHO member countries to develop policies and plans for the prevention and control of violence against women and the launching of the integrated approach the following year. From the beginning, PAHO and WHO have been at the forefront of building up the evidence base on the magnitude and nature of intimate partner violence and sexual violence, through studies such as the Critical Path (Sagot 2000) and the WHO Multi-Country Study on Women's Health and Domestic Violence (WHO 2002). This proactive resolve is well captured in WHO's recently launched *World Report on Health and Violence.* In the report's preface, the Organization's Director-General, Gro Harlem Brundtland, notes: "The report also challenges us in many respects. It forces us beyond our notions of what is acceptable and comfortable—to challenge notions that acts of violence are simply matters of family privacy, individual choice, or inevitable facets of life" (WHO 2002).

The search for effective and long-lasting solutions, from interventions for primary prevention to caring for the victims and survivors of violence, is ongoing. However, in terms of "what works," the experiences are still limited and scattered and often not well documented and disseminated. The efforts by the Pan American Health Organization to document its experience in Central America in this book is therefore an important contribution to this field.

It seems obvious to point out that when developing responses to gender-based violence, it is necessary to take into account the particular locale and the resources available, the prevailing social norms and laws, and the characteristics of the health, legal, and other sectors. No one model "fits all," and each intervention will need to be adapted to the specific context (social, cultural, political) in which it is being applied. However, many of the lessons learned from experiences like the ones described in this book may have wider applicability, in spite of coming from one region of the world, and could serve in many respects to guide responses in other settings. This chapter discusses the wider applicability of the approach used by PAHO and its partners in Latin America to other settings.

THE PAHO APPROACH: NEW LOCALES, NEW POSSIBILITIES

PAHO's work on gender-based violence started with the Critical Path Study described in Chapter Two. The importance of this study was that it documented and provided the first in-depth understanding of what happened to women once they broke their silence and actively sought help: from state services, church and schools in their community, and even neighbors and family members. Acquiring this type of information and understanding, which could be obtained in different ways and at times by adapting and even simplifying the methodology, is an important basis upon which to develop interventions. As we have seen, the results provide critical insight into the nature and variety of roadblocks and other obstacles women commonly face in their search for care and support. In addition, the study suggested that for every woman who does seek help, there are many, many more whose suffering remains invisible. How do we reach this group, and how do we encourage these women so that they can transform their lives and end the violence they face daily? Improving the response of the existing services–formal and informal– is the most obvious and logical starting point for this change to take place.

The review of the PAHO approach to violence against women; specifically, its work in diverse communities across Central America, as described in Section II of this book, revealed key characteristics that succeeded in finding roots despite the peculiarities of geography, social and cultural beliefs, and political structures. On the contrary, these qualities suggest the approach's relevance and potential adaptability to other corners of the world where women do not yet have access to services and systems that might provide recognition, care, and support. As other communities contemplate taking the first step toward responding to these women, they might wish to keep in mind the approach's overarching commonalities, presented below, and find them of use in localizing the strategy in new settings:

(1) **The approach is flexible and non-prescriptive.** In each PAHO project community, the principal stakeholders mutually identified the specific approach to be taken, which were the best institutions and/or departments to guide the process, and who were the most relevant partners. While there was one common overriding goal and similar accompanying objectives, there was no drive to impose a single generic model on all settings in the seven project countries.

(2) **The approach calls for action at several levels.** Project participants soon recognized that simultaneous action at multiple levels offers the best possibility for a "successful" response to violence. Specifically, these levels are: (a) the macro level of national policies; (b) in programs of different public sectors, with a focus on the health sector; and (c) at the level of the community. Concrete actions must be developed at all three of these levels, and action at each level serves to synergistically support and reinforce the response in the other levels.

(3) **A multisectoral approach achieves the best results.** The need for a plurality of disciplines and fields of expertise–health, education, law enforcement, the courts system–coming to bear on the issue of violence is now well recognized and documented. Yet the forging of this primordial dynamic has been–so far, at least–perhaps the most elusive of all goals to achieve and maintain. This might be because, in responding to violence, there is no one obvious sector to take the lead. Which force becomes the standard-bearer, so to speak, will vary in different settings and is often related to a key personality who is willing to move the issue forward. In some Latin American countries, it has been the legal and judicial sector which has come to the forefront, while in others it has been the health sector, and in still others, it has been the office of women's affairs.

In the PAHO Central America project, priority was given to the health sector, as the natural counterpart of PAHO. Regardless of which sector takes the lead, a public health approach nonetheless seeks to ensure that all sectors are engaged, work collaboratively, and that their roles are well specified and mutually reinforcing. A plan of action delineating the specific role and functions of each sector can help to clarify and minimize "territorial disputes." Resource allocation at the national and/or local levels will also need to reflect adequately the role of each sector.

(4) Partnerships and networks provide the necessary underpinning. In all the PAHO project settings, women's organizations dedicated to ending gender-based violence were involved and played a key role in the development of the response. This point cannot be emphasized enough. It is thanks to the persistent and highly energized efforts of women's organizations and the women's rights movement that the issue of gender-based violence is on the global political agenda today. At a time when neither the world's interest in, nor the strategic resources for, advocacy work against violence were available, these organizations struggled unrelentingly, often despite meager funding sources, to provide a response to and support for women living in violent situations. It is critical that they do not become marginalized at this juncture, but rather that their expertise and commitment be permanently harnessed in the creation of new and broader responses by governments and other actors to a problem that persists in nearly every society around the world.

Partnerships and multisectoral action at the community level require time, energy, commitment, and resources. The development of networks, as has been achieved by PAHO and its collaborators, is only the first step in the process. One of the important lessons learned is that once a network is established, additional input and support are needed to ensure that the network remains active. Developing clear objectives and monitoring the impact of the network's

activities are equally important. Globally, there is a need to evaluate more systematically the impact and benefits of both formal and informal networks to address gender-based violence, such as was done with those created by the Central American project.

GALVANIZING THE HEALTH SECTOR RESPONSE

A particular objective of the initiative to stop GBV, and of the work of PAHO and WHO specifically, is to strengthen the health sector's response, keeping in mind the need for collaboration within this sector and with other sectors. The Critical Path study provided countless descriptions of inconsequential, non-supportive, and even damaging encounters between women and health personnel. Thus, a focus on improving the health sector response was well justified, not only because this government entity is the natural counterpart to PAHO and WHO, but because it is the one sector which women are most likely to come into contact with at some point in their lives.

As has been discussed elsewhere (García-Moreno 2002), the health sector has a fundamental role to play in violence prevention and in caring for women affected by this problem. A key function lies in the identification of women seeking health services for whom violence may be an underlying risk factor. A supportive encounter with the health sector, it is argued, may enable a woman to recognize the problem if she has not yet done so, may encourage her to seek help, and may help her to access care, treatment, and support from other community sources. Asking a woman about violence can shed light on the underlying causes for the clinical problems she identifies as the formal reason for her consultation, and, to the degree to which she is ready to talk, lead to a more accurate diagnosis, better targeted treatment, and the identification of other appropriate community resources and services as needed. Knowledge that a woman is suffering from violence can also contribute to the prevention of further episodes and to potential morbidity and mortality from this cause.

For all this to happen, however, the health encounter needs to take place in a confidential and caring setting, with a provider who is sensitive, nonjudgmental, and willing to spend sufficient time to provide the support and care needed. In turn, health providers must be equipped with the knowledge and skills that will allow them not only to identify women in violent situations, but to provide them with the subsequent treatment, care, and referrals needed.

As the experience of PAHO and others (Guedes 2002 et al.) has shown, enabling the health sector to respond appropriately to GBV, and sustaining this response, is not an easy task. This is because concerted, interconnected action at different levels of the public health hierarchy are key to this sustainability. Health policies, norms, and protocols at the national, local, and facility level provide the necessary blueprint for the development and implementation of training and intervention programs. As we have seen in the various countries, no one approach or entry point exists; rather, there are different options, and in each case the best choice depends on the availability of a range of resources, including funds, staff, and commitment. Some of the key elements of the health sector's work, as well as the areas that were identified as needing strengthening in the PAHO experience, are discussed below. These observations and experiences may be useful to others in addressing GBV issues in their own communities.

TRAINING OF HEALTH PERSONNEL

Training is critical to developing and sustaining a high-quality, long-term health sector response to gender-based violence. Reviews of training programs on violence against women for health providers show that in many cases these are not satisfactory and the content and quality are variable and inconsistent (Davidson et al. 2001). Many of the programs tend to be of limited duration, and while they may raise awareness of the problem, they may not always provide sufficient skills or address providers' values and attitudes that impact on their ability to respond to the problem. Also, they tend to focus on the individual provider and rarely address the structural or institutional context within which the provider's work takes place (García-Moreno 2002).

One of the limitations of many training programs has been that they become an end in themselves, with little attention to the structural and other transformations that need to accompany training. The PAHO approach included an emphasis on training, involving the technical input, support, and participation of ministries of health and other local entities. Numerous health providers (and other community service providers) have been trained throughout the life of the project. There has been, however, little systematic evaluation of this training and its impact.

The PAHO experience also has led to the development of a broad range of training tools and materials, many of which are targeted to specific groups, including indigenous cultures, schoolteachers, children, and men, and which take into account local customs and values. But might not this body of local inspiration find a larger audience? Perhaps at this stage it would be helpful to review the wealth of what is available, cull the best examples, and determine the keys to their impact. While there may be a need for local specificity in the development of these materials, it is also important to avoid reinventing the wheel and duplicating efforts. A comprehensive review of which training tools and approaches have worked best in the different Central American settings would be of great value to the participating countries and stimulate new interest in larger circles beyond.

While the PAHO review did not include a quantitative assessment of the outcomes and impact of the various health sector training programs that have been developed as part of the project, it nonetheless provides indications for further work by highlighting the numerous lessons learned and key ingredients which could lead to a more lasting impact of training activities in the future. These are briefly outlined below:

(1) **A systems approach may increase impact.** An approach that takes into account the overall system rather than focusing only on the health provider has the potential to have more impact. Otherwise, providers may find themselves unable to implement changes, even with the sufficient knowledge and motivation to do so. In this project, training of providers was supported by variable degrees of institutional change and the development of norms and protocols to guide providers, and in some cases, administrators as well.

(2) **Universal screening is not always the golden standard.** "Universal screening," i.e., asking all women coming through a health service about exposure to violence, is usually taken as the golden standard. Yet there may be situations in which asking women may not be feasible or cannot be done in a way that ensures confidentiality. In this situation, providing the woman with basic information in portable form, such as a leaflet or brochure, regarding services at the provider's facility or elsewhere in the community, may be more useful and less likely to cause harm. To be effective and to "do no harm," universal screening needs to be supported by intensive provider training, system changes, and the availability of care protocols and norms, with ongoing monitoring of their implementation and of the screening process's impact on the lives of the women themselves. The guiding principle of any health service response must be to "do no harm," and this should orient and inform the introduction of changes in the health sector, so that while universal screening may remain the long-term objective, there may be other steps that are necessary before a health service can introduce this in a systematic manner.

(3) **Mere identification is not enough.** Identifying women who are living with violence is really only the first step. An adequate response is necessary, and it is suggested that as a minimum this should include: appropriate care and treatment, assessment of immediate danger, the provision of information on or referral to existing services, counseling and developing a safety plan with the woman, and providing follow-up and support. However, special challenges arise when there are few or no other services to which women may be referred and providers have limited resources for follow-up and support. This is particularly true in small towns or remote rural areas, as we have seen in the case of Central America. There is a much higher risk that these women will fall through the cracks and never be heard from again, as we have also seen. In this situation, other strategies need to be identified, during the initial consultation, always keeping the women's safety and well-being as the paramount consideration.

(4) Horizontal versus vertical integration of violence programs: which works best? Integrating violence concerns across different health programs appears to be more useful than addressing violence as a separate vertical program. Several entry points exist in the organization of health services, as was shown in the Central American project. In some countries, violence work took place from within reproductive health services, while in others, violence activities formed part of mental health services. In still other countries, accident and emergency departments have served as the starting points, as have primary outpatient services (García-Moreno 2002). Generally, however, reproductive health services are more widely available– even in low resource settings–and those most likely to be used by women–ill and healthy–at some point in their lives, thereby providing a natural entry point for addressing GBV. However, the best location will depend on the specific circumstances of each locale and its available resources, which would include the existence of a supportive administrative environment and policies. In the Central American review, overall it appeared that reproductive health services were most likely to have the basic resources and support mechanisms necessary to address violence, particularly compared to mental health services. In an ideal context, all health services for women should incorporate GBV considerations into their work, so that these considerations are integrated horizontally across the spectrum of health services offerings. Inter-programmatic coordination is a vital element to ensure that the women receive continuity in care and consistent messages about their problems, no matter which type of health service they seek.

(5) Caregivers need emotional support. For those on the front lines of response,

caring for women suffering from violence can be a very draining experience. While there is general agreement that caregivers should be provided with emotional support systems, as we have seen, this rarely occurs in reality. The valuable service provided by health professionals to their clients–at times even life-saving–as well as the mental and physical toll it claims on these providers, requires more recognition and compensation. Resources need to be allocated to offset the potentially harmful effects to providers' health and well-being by creating structured time and space mechanisms in which caregivers can share their experiences, emotions, and needs.

(6) The approach to GBV should be holistic. At times, there is a tendency towards a fragmentation in response to different forms of violence, meaning that the treatment for the physical, sexual, and psychological/emotional sequelae are sometimes separated (or some are not addressed at all). A holistic approach would integrate the health response to these different manifestations regardless of the victim's relationship to the perpetrator (intimate partner, other family member or relative, acquaintance, or stranger). In practice, programs have tended to focus on only two types of violence–that by intimate partners living in the same household (sometimes also called "domestic" or "intrafamily" violence) and sexual violence, usually perpetrated by strangers. Response to the latter has tended to emphasize the importance of the victim submitting to a forensic medical examination, sometimes to the detriment of (and separately from) the health care response.

It is important to be aware of the various types of health and other needs arising from these different situations of violence. For example, a single event of rape by a stranger or a gang rape gives rise to particular health care needs, including that of a forensic medical examination. These needs are likely to be different to those of a woman suffering from ongoing abuse by an intimate partner occurring over many years. Intimate partner abuse oftentimes escalates in frequency and/or intensity, so the risks may vary as well at different times. Yet it is not realistic, particularly in resource-poor settings, to have separate services for different types of violence. In many places, care and support, regardless of the type of abuse, are likely to be provided by the same practitioner. The nature of professional training and of the specific norms and protocols, therefore, needs to address the local range of needs and situations as much as possible. In some settings, for example, specific forms of violence such as dowry-related or female genital cutting may need to be included in training on gender-based violence. One of the lessons learned was that when setting up GBV services, the most effective strategy is to integrate rather than fragment the response to violence's many forms. Based on this, PAHO project participants in the future plan to expand work beyond the current focus of intimate partner abuse to such areas as sexual abuse, including child sexual abuse.

(7) Documentation and follow-up are central elements to the health sector response. It is important for health services personnel to record accurately and completely the information on abuse they gather from their clients. It is equally important to ensure the confidentiality of this data and that there are mechanisms to protect against its misuse. The availability of accurate and complete documentation could help ensure better response, care, and follow-up. However, the "rules of the game" in information-sharing across sectors (for example, between doctors and police officials) remain largely a grey area, and other sectors sometimes secure access to sensitive information without the consent of the affected woman. Also, if the same woman requests services in different areas within the heath sector, problems often result that could perhaps be improved with better record-keeping. Inconsistencies in health information intake and management were identified as one of the weakest components in the PAHO study, despite the importance of this information when developing new interventions. There needs to be greater clarity about what data need to be collected, by whom, and for what purpose. Record-keeping and data-gathering are most likely to be done correctly when those doing this understand and see the value of the process—particularly its usefulness in monitoring performance and impact (both their own and the health service's in general).

THE HEALTH SECTOR AND THE COMMUNITY

The following sections address the health sector's interaction with other sectors and entities in the community and present observations based on the Central American experience with potential wider applicability to other GBV programs:

(1) The health sector should be proactive in raising community awareness about women and violence issues and GBV prevention. The work inside the health sector can be greatly enhanced by an advocacy and communication strategy that raises local awareness of the problem and informs the general public about the availability of services. During the Central American review, health professionals noted that many of the posters and brochures currently used in their clinics had not been specifically developed for health care settings. Furthermore, workers at various points suggested that ministries of health and PAHO develop a regionwide health promotion campaign targeting GBV and encouraging women to talk to their providers about violence. Clearly, such a campaign–in the Americas and other WHO regions– could gain resonance from the participation of other sector partners, if the messages crafted present a unified voice against violence. Therefore, each partner's contribution must be a clear and accurate reflection of this sector's field of expertise, and at the same time buttress messages by others. This same dynamic applies at the local level, where it is even more critical for the sector services to create and sustain linkages and present coherent messages that address the gamut of GBV issues–personal health and well-being, the family, available support systems, and legal rights and protections.

(2) **The legal and health interface requires clearer definition.** Mandatory reporting, i.e., the requirement that health workers provide information to law enforcement officials regarding all patients they suspect to be victims of domestic violence, deserves special mention in this chapter, as it remains a controversial issue. The requirement originated with the need to report child abuse, given the status of children as minors in need of state protection. In the case of adult women, however, many women's group advocates–and sometimes the women themselves–consider that they should be able to decide freely whether to seek protection or not, rather than having this imposed upon them by the judgement of others. Further, some studies indicate that mandatory reporting may pose a threat to the safety of women in abusive relationships and may create barriers to their seeking help or talking with health providers about their problem (Rodríguez 1998).

In at least three of the Central American countries participating in the PAHO project, mandatory reporting for intimate partner violence against women has been instituted. PAHO and health policymakers in the Americas will need to close ranks and present a clearer position on this in the future, in keeping with the guiding principles of "doing no harm" and respect for women's autonomy and decision-making capacity. As new programs emerge in other parts of the world, these players, as well, will need to carefully examine the pros and cons of different government policies, such as mandatory reporting, and, in particular, determine their impact on women's lives and safety.

(3) **GBV monitoring and surveillance are particularly weak when compared to other health issues.** Central to violence prevention is the ongoing availability to gather and disseminate accurate information about the types and amount of violence in a particular location, factors that are associated with it, and the consequences of that violence. This information is essential for heightening the problem's visibility–particularly the significance of its contribution to morbidity and mortality statistics–but also for informed policy formation, strategic decision-making, and the appropriate allocation of health resources. Surveillance on violence against women poses particular challenges, as noted by Campbell (Campbell 2000) and discussed in Chapter Five.

One serious weakness identified in the PAHO project was the fact that information systems for tracking violence were often developed independently of the norms and protocols for its treatment. Despite having received training on information-gathering and recording, if professionals do not possess the proper skills and techniques for asking about violence or the institutional environment is not conducive to this process, the necessary data may not be collected or might not be reliable. This may not only be harmful for the affected women, but also creates the false impression that violence is not an issue of social and political concern in the community. Furthermore, as Chapter Five pointedly notes, information-gathering by health professionals and others presents the ethical imperative to provide care and services in return.

When introducing a system to record GBV-related information cases, its effectiveness is directly proportional to its compatibility and uniformity with systems in other areas within the same country, at the very least. Ideally, however, global standards, such as the WHO Injury Surveillance system (WHO 2001) and the International Classification of Diseases (ICD-10) categories should be followed whenever possible.

A minimum standard set of information—the type of violence (physical, sexual, emotional, etc.), and the age and sex of the victim, as well as the age and relationship of the perpetrator to the victim—should be universally uniform to enable comparisons between systems. Additionally, data on violence presented centrally should always be disaggregated by sex and age.

(4) Community networks and support groups for violence survivors provide a springboard for solidarity and action.

A key element of the PAHO approach is its emphasis on the creation of dynamic community networks for the prevention of violence. The positive work and achievements of these networks in all the PAHO project settings attest to the almost limitless opportunities for sustainable and locally developed responses with which the larger community can develop a sense of identity and ownership. The impact of women's groups and well-known, committed local leaders and decision-makers has already been noted. The combined synergy of these and other high-profile grassroots players has contributed perhaps more than any other factor to the transformation of social norms that once unquestionably viewed gender-based violence as a private family matter off-limits to public scrutiny and preventive action.

In many of the PAHO project communities, support groups for violence survivors offered positive reinforcement and practical strategies to women in abusive relatioships. In other settings, however, the results of similar endeavors were mixed and inconclusive. There appears to be no "magic formula" beyond the personal skills and deftness of the group facilitator in engaging the participants in finding workable solutions to their situations, regardless of that leader's specific background or training. These groups are attractive in this sense, because they can provide a vibrant, ongoing source of support for women in resource-poor settings, with a minimum of investment from the "formal" sector. At the same time, they create the potential for collective action and the challenging of public perceptions about the inescapability of violence. It is important to explore these type of initiatives further and evaluate more systematically the structure and components of the most successful among them, how they have ensured continuity and sustainability over time, and what types of support (institutional, financial, training, etc.) they feel have most contributed to their effectiveness.

FINAL WORDS

This chapter seeks to highlight how the groundbreaking work of PAHO and its many collaborators in Central America can find new roots in other communities throughout the Americas and the world. The authors of this book have followed the development of the Critical Path study and subsequent project review closely and have shared their insights so that others might see what has worked and what has not worked in the various settings. The lessons learned presented herein, while perhaps bearing the sociocultural and political idiosyncrasies of their geographical birthplace, nonetheless afford glimpses of local adaptability in communities everywhere in the world where women remain the invisible and choiceless victims of violence.

World human rights activist and Nobel laureate Nelson Mandela recently referred to the "legacy of day-to-day, individual suffering", observing that:

> This suffering . . . is a legacy that reproduces itself, as new generations learn from the violence of generations past, as victims learn from victimizers, and as the social conditions that nurture violence are allowed to continue. No country, no city, no community is immune. But neither are we powerless against it.

Instead, he notes with firm conviction,

> Violence can be prevented. . . . In my own country and around the world, we have shining examples of how violence has been countered. Governments, communities, and individuals can make a difference. [1]

Mandela's final statement is perhaps the most important lesson learned by PAHO and its partners in Central America (and the Andean countries, as well). Governments, communities, and the courageous victims of violence themselves have taken the first steps that in the future will enable these women to live lives free from violence and fear. Their collective achievements are a call to action to others. For if the roots of violence remain hidden behind closed doors, the family—the nucleus for the cross-generational imprinting of human values and ideals—is irrevocably damaged, and society's wellspring of aspirations for future transformation and cleansing is rendered barren. This specter should compel even the most sceptical and resistant to urgent action. ⬎

---

[1] *Excerpts from Foreword of the* World Report on Violence and Health *(WHO 2002)*

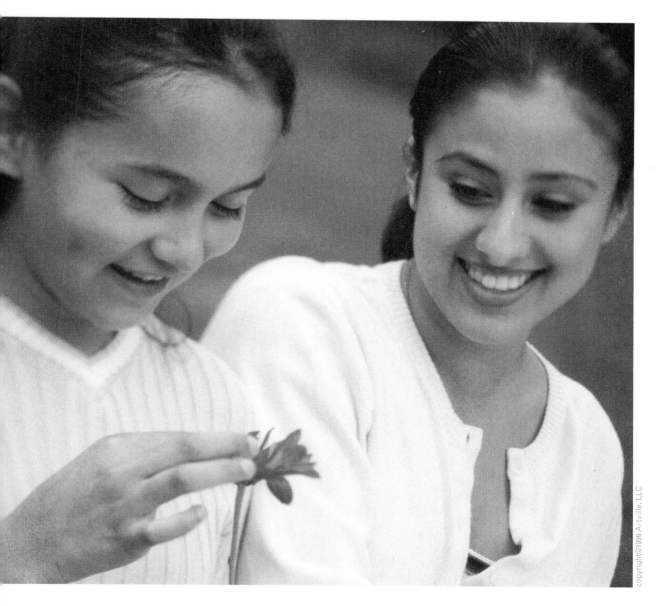

GBV RESOURCES SECTION

The following resource materials have been compiled as a service to our readers. Resources are organized reverse-chronologically and alphabetically. Those resources only available in Spanish or not available online are so indicated. The section groupings are:

I. PAHO (Women, Health, and Development Program/HDW) and WHO Materials
II. Program for Appropriate Technology in Health (PATH) Materials
III. Centers for Disease Control and Prevention (CDC) Materials
IV. Other Background Materials
V. Training Manuals and Guides
VI. Conventions and Declarations
VII. Internet/Web Resources

I. PAHO AND WHO MATERIALS

⟡ HDW Gender and Health Fact Sheets

HDW/PAHO publishes a monthly fact sheet in English and Spanish on a current theme in gender equity and health. Topics related to GBV include:
- Men's Role in Gender-Based Violence, 2002
- Social Responses to Gender-Based Violence, 2002
- Trafficking of Women and Children for Sexual Exploitation in the Americas, 2001
- Domestic Violence during Pregnancy, 2000
- Health Workers and Gender-Based Violence, 2000

http://www.paho.org/english/hdp/hdw/factsheets.htm

⟡ WHO Multi-Country Study on Women's Health and Domestic Violence
World Health Organization, 2002.

An introductory brochure to the study, which is policy- and action-oriented and is being carried out in partnership with research institutions and/or national ministries and women's organizations working on issues related to violence in eight countries.
http://whqlibdoc.who.int/hq/2002/WHO_FCH_GWH_02.2.pdf

⟡ World Report on Violence and Health. *World Health Organization, 2002.*

Chapter 4 of the report discusses intimate partner violence, and Chapter 6 discusses sexual violence. http://www5.who.int/violence_injury_prevention/main.cfm?p=0000000682

⟡ Interagency Manual on Reproductive Health in Refugee Situations: Sexual and Gender-Based Violence. *World Health Organization, 2001.*

Chapter 4 focuses on sexual violence against women. Most reported cases of sexual violence among refugees involve female victims and male perpetrators. It is acknowledged that men and young boys may also be vulnerable to sexual violence.
http://www.who.int/reproductivehealth/publications/interagency_manual_on_RH_in_refugee_situations/ch4.pdf

⟡ The Integrated Model of Care of Intra-Family Violence. *Pan American Health Organization, 2001*

In the last few years in Central America, a series of efforts have contributed to ensure that all seven countries recognize intra-family violence as a public health concern deserving immediate attention. As a result, countries have put into place legislation and committed human and financial resources designed to facilitate the operation and consolidation of a model of integral care to respond to intra-family violence.
http://www.paho.org/English/HDP/HDW/integratedmodel.pdf

⟡ Symposium 2001 Final Report: Gender-Based Violence, Health, and Rights in the Americas. *Pan American Health Organization, 2001.*

From 4–7 June 2001, the Symposium brought together representatives from the ministries of health, women's NGOs, civil society, and U.N. agencies from 30 countries as well as international donor agencies to identify priorities and formulate strategies for strengthening the response of the health sector to GBV.
http://www.paho.org/English/HDP/HDW/Symposium2001FinalReport.htm

➔ *La ruta crítica que siguen las mujeres afectadas por la violencia intrafamiliar.*
Pan American Health Organization, 2000.
Translated into English as: *Domestic Violence: Women's Way Out.*
This publication demonstrates that intra-family violence is a complex problem which requires coordinated and intersectoral solutions involving the participation of both the State and civil society.
Spanish: http://www.paho.org/Spanish/HDP/HDW/rutacritica.htm
English: http://www.paho.org/English/HDP/HDW/womenswayout.htm

➔ **Violence against Women: WHO Fact Sheet No. 239.**
World Health Organization, 2000.
Violence against women and girls is a major health and human rights concern. While violence has severe health consequences for the affected, it is a social problem that warrants an immediate coordinated response from multiple sectors.
http://www.who.int/inf-fs/en/fact239.html

➔ **Violence against Women and HIV/AIDS: Setting the Research Agenda.**
World Health Organization, 2000.
This meeting report is divided into three main sections. The first section contains a summary of each presentation. The second section summarizes the discussion, and the third details the recommendations and conclusions from the meeting (held 23–25 October 2000).
http://www5.who.int/violence_injury_prevention/download.cfm?id=0000000151

➔ **Annotated Bibliography on Violence against Women: A Health and Human Rights Concern.** *World Health Organization, 1999.*
Commissioned by the Global Commission on Women's Health. Prepared by Rights and Humanity in collaboration with the WHO Women's Health and Development Unit and the Global Commission on Women's Health.
http://whqlibdoc.who.int/hq/1999/WHO_CHS_GCWH_99.2.pdf

➔ **Gender and Public Health Series**
This series published by PAHO contains the following GBV-related topics:
Nº1   Battered Women: A Working Guide for Crisis Intervention, 1999
Nº7   Helping Ourselves to Help Others: Self-Care Guide for Those Who Work in the Field of Family Violence, 1999. http://www.paho.org/English/HDP/HDW/gphseries.htm

➔ **Putting Women First: Ethical and Safety Recommendations for Research on Domestic Violence against Women.**
World Health Organization, 1999.
Research on violence against women raises important ethical and methodological challenges. Researching abuse is not like other areas of investigation—the nature of the topic means that issues of safety, confidentiality, and interviewer skills and training are even more important than in other forms of research.
http://www5.who.int/violence_injury_prevention/download.cfm?id=0000000130

➤ **Violence against Women: A Priority Health Issue Information Pack.**
World Health Organization, 1997.
The package focuses on violence in families, rape, and sexual assault, violence against women in situations of conflict and displacement, as well as violence against the girl child. The consequences of violence on women's health and the role that public health workers can play in multisectoral efforts to end the violence are explored. http://www5.who.int/violence_injury_prevention/download.cfm?id=0000000154

II. PATH MATERIALS

➤ **Reproductive Health and Rights: Reaching the Hardly Reached.** *2002.*
This publication is a compendium of articles that highlight the negative impact that marginal status has on the health and well-being of various vulnerable groups. Various aspects of gender-based violence are presented and included in several articles. http://www.path.org/materials-details.php?id=503

➤ **Violence against Women: Effects on Reproductive Health.**
Outlook, Volume 20, #1, 2002.
This report presents an overview of violence from a public health perspective. It describes the effects of violence on women's reproductive health. The report provides examples from research and successful programs and explores how the health sector can take an active role in the prevention and treatment of violence against women. http://www.path.org/resources/pub_outlook.htm

➤ **Reproductive Health, Gender, and Human Rights: A Dialogue.** *2001.*
This publication is a collection of articles by public health and human rights experts who examine both the common interests and significant differences that the two perspectives bring to reproductive health issues. http://www.path.org/materials-details.php?id=427

III. CDC MATERIALS

➤ **Extent, Nature, and Consequences of Intimate Partner Violence:**
Findings from the National Violence against Women Survey. *2000.*
This National Institute of Justice research report presents findings from a survey of 8,000 U.S. women and 8,000 U.S. men about their experiences as victims of intimate partner violence (rape, physical assault, and stalking). http://www.ojp.usdoj.gov/nij/pubs-sum/181867.htm

➤ **The Screen Show on Intimate Partner Violence during Pregnancy.**
American College of Obstetricians and Gynecologists and CDC, 2000.
A training tool to help increase clinicians' understanding of the important role they can play to identify, prevent, and reduce intimate partner violence. The content of the screen show is supplemented by a bibliography, references to several protocols for screening, and organization resource lists. http://www.cdc.gov/nccdphp/drh/violence/ipvdp.htm

→ **Violence and Reproductive Health.**
Maternal and Child Health Journal, Volume 4, #2, 2000.
This special issue looks at such topics as screening practices for abuse during prenatal visits; the role of reproductive health care services; the relationship between sexual abuse and sexual risk; and women, violence, and HIV.
http://www.cdc.gov/nccdphp/drh/wh_viol_mchjv4n2.htm

→ **Building Data Systems for Monitoring and Responding to Violence against Women.** *1998.*
This report provides recommendations regarding public health surveillance and research on violence against women developed during a workshop held 29–30 October 1998.
http://www.cdc.gov/mmwr/preview/mmwrhtml/rr4911a1.htm

→ **Intimate Partner Violence and Sexual Assault:**
A Guide to Training Materials and Programs for Health Care Providers. *1998.*
A guide to help individuals and organizations find appropriate materials for group or self-training. http://www.cdc.gov/ncipc/pub-res/ipvasa.htm

IV. OTHER BACKGROUND MATERIALS

→ **Supplemental Issue on The Role of Health Professionals in Addressing Violence against Women.** *International Journal of Gynecology and Obstetrics, 78 (Supplement 1), 2002.*
This issue includes articles on violence against women and Brazilian health care policies; American College of Obstetricians and Gynecologists: responding to violence against women; and a global overview of gender-based violence, among others.
Full text available via ScienceDirect: http://www.sciencedirect.com

→ **Gender Dimensions of Alcohol and Alcohol-Related Problems in Latin America and the Caribbean.** *World Bank, 2001.*
This report examines the gender dimensions of alcohol consumption and alcohol-related problems in Latin America and the Caribbean. Its principal findings are: (1) men bear most of the burden of alcohol-related diseases; (2) alcohol plays an important role in instigating unsafe sex practices and violent behaviors, including domestic violence; and (3) men are more likely than women to drink alcohol heavily and excessively, and drinking norms influence these gender differences in alcohol consumption.
http://lnweb18.worldbank.org/external
/lac/lac.nsf/Sectors/Gender/1664193800FD252185256B75006A0324?OpenDocument

→ **Picturing a Life Free of Violence: Media and Communication Strategies to End Violence against Women.** *United Nations Development Fund for Women (UNIFEM), 2001.*
This report showcases a variety of media and communications strategies to be used to end violence against women. The report is a collaboration between UNIFEM and the Media Materials Clearinghouse of the Johns Hopkins University Center for Communications Programs. http://www.unifem.undp.org/resources/freeofviolence/index.html

⇢ **Researching Domestic Violence against Women: Methodological and Ethical Considerations.** (Ellsberg M, Heise L, Agurto S, Peña R, Winkvist A.) *Studies in Family Planning 32(1), Population Council, 2001.*

This report compares the findings of three population-based studies on violence against women in Nicaragua. The report examines the differences among the results and the possible effects of methodological factors on underreporting and validity. (Not available online.)

⇢ **Silence for the Sake of Harmony: Domestic Violence and Health in Central Java, Indonesia.** *CHN-RL GMU, Rifka Annisa Women's Crisis Center, Umeå University, Women's Health Exchange and PATH. 2001.*

This publication presents research on the prevalence and incidence of violence against women in Indonesia. It presents the methodology used and the research results and concludes with recommendations. (Available through PATH.)

⇢ **Domestic Violence against Women and Girls.** *Innocenti Digest 6, United Nations Children's Fund (UNICEF), 2000.*

This study on domestic violence describes the powerlessness of women in situations of violence and notes that up to half of the world's female population may be victimized by those closest to them at some time in their lives. Within this context, issues related to intimate partner violence take on added urgency because of the rapid spread of the AIDS virus in many parts of the world. http://www.unicef-icdc.org/publications/pdf/digest6e.pdf

⇢ **Dying of Sadness: Sexual Violence and the HIV Epidemic.** *United Nations Development Program (UNDP), 2000.*

This preliminary overview of available literature suggests that, within the context of gender and the HIV epidemic, sexual violence is a complex phenomenon with multiple determinants, consequences, and manifestations. http://www.undp.org/seped/publications/dyingofsadness.pdf

⇢ **Justice, Change, and Human Rights: International Research and Responses to Domestic Violence.** *Center for Development and Population Activities, 2000.*

This paper employs both a human rights and a development framework to identify the limitations and strengths of each approach for understanding and responding to domestic violence, as well as to clarify the links that need to be made between the frameworks. http://www.cedpa.org/publications/pdf/violenceprowid.pdf

⇢ **With an End in Sight.** *UNIFEM, 2000.*

A publication that documents seven important programs dedicated to ending violence against women in Bosnia and Herzegovina, Cambodia, Honduras, India, Kenya, Nigeria, and the West Bank and Gaza. http://www.unifem.undp.org/resources/tfbook/index.html

→ **Ending Violence against Women.**
(Heise L, Ellsberg M, Gottemoeller M.) *Population Reports 27(4),*
Johns Hopkins University Center for Communication Programs, 1999.
In-depth study by the Johns Hopkins School of Public Health and the Center for Health and
Gender Equity. Based on over 50 population-based surveys and more than 500 studies of
domestic violence, the report finds that by far the greatest risk of violence comes not from
strangers, but from male family members, including husbands.
In English: http://www.jhuccp.org/pr/l11edsum.stm
In Spanish: http://www.jhuccp.org/prs/sl11edsum.stm

→ **Violence against Women, Gender, and Health Equity.**
Harvard Center for Population and Development Studies, 1999.
This paper starts with a broad definition of violence against women and then focuses on
domestic and sexual violence in particular. It provides an overview of the magnitude of
domestic and sexual violence against women and of its various consequences including
those involving health for women and their children.
http://www.hsph.harvard.edu/Organizations /healthnet/HUpapers/gender/garcia.html

→ **The Facts about Gender-Based Violence.**
International Planned Parenthood Federation, 1998.
This report provides a definition of gender-based violence and includes statistics on its
worldwide magnitude. It also details the different forms of violence that women face every
day ranging from sexual harassment to female genital mutilation and rape.
http://www.ippf.org/resource/gbv/ma98/1.htm

→ **The Intimate Enemy: Gender Violence and Reproductive Health.**
The Panos Institute, 1998.
The report shows how local communities around the world are providing medical, legal,
and counseling services for victims and lobbying for changes in laws and customs to address
the problem head-on. http://www.panos.org.uk/briefing/genviol.htm

→ **The Nicaraguan Network of Women against Violence:**
Using Research and Action for Change.
(Ellsberg M, Liljestrand J, Winkvist A.) *Reproductive Health Matters #10. 1997.*
This report examines the anti-violence movement in Nicaragua, which began in the 1980s
and has been led by the Nicaraguan Network of Women against Violence. It outlines the
various strategies used to advocate for the inclusion of domestic violence on the country's
national political agenda. (Not available online.)

→ **Gender-Based Violence: A Human Rights Issue.**
Mujer y Desarrollo Series #16. Economic Comisión for Latin America and the Caribbean, 1996.
The study explores the various forms of GBV and how growing awareness of the phenomenon
in recent years has led to the establishment of new institutions and the adoption of legislative
amendments, which in turn have served as a focal point for collective action by women.
http://www.eclac.cl/publicaciones/UnidadMujer/7/lcl957/lcl957i.pdf

V. TRAINING MANUALS AND GUIDES

✦ *Violencia domestica: Modelo de intervención en unidades de salud*
[Domestic Violence: Model of Intervention in Public Health Units]. (Volumes 1-3).
Inter-American Development Bank, 2002.
This manual is a guide for the development of multidisciplinary networks for the detection and care of intra-family violence against women from the perspective of the health sector. Available only in Spanish. (Not available online.)

✦ **A Practical Approach to Gender-Based Violence:**
A Program Guide for Health Care Providers and Managers.
United Nations Population Fund, 2001.
This publication contains practical steps needed to integrate gender-based violence into reproductive health facilities. It is also meant to help a wider range of readers understand the interrelationships between reproductive and sexual health and violence.
http://www.unfpa.org/publications/gender.pdf

✦ **Confronting Chronic Neglect: The Education and Training of Health Professionals on Family Violence.** *U.S. Institute of Medicine, 2001.*
The book identifies the gaps which exist in current training and the challenges identified by health professionals in their attempts to address violence. It also sets out priority areas for future training efforts and presents a number of recommendations to guide those efforts.
http://www.nap.edu/books/0309074312/html/

✦ *Manual para el abordaje de la violencia contra la mujer*
[Manual for Approaching the Issue of Violence against Women].
Mujer Vamos Adelante and CICAM, 2001.
The primary objective of this manual is to make women themselves aware of their rights, specifically their right to live free from violence. The publication is divided into the following sections: a review of international human rights declarations and instruments; the Guatemalan legal/constitutional context; what is violence against women?; where does violence happen and who perpetrates it?; what forms does violence take?; why should you denounce violence?; who can denounce violence?; how can you denounce violence?; what is the role of the public sector?; what is the role of the police?; what is the role of the judiciary?; how is violence registered?; and what happens after you denounce violence. Available only in Spanish. (Not available online.)

✦ **Tools for Providers Working with Victims of Gender-Based Violence.**
International Planned Parenthood Federation, 2001.
The tools in this publication were developed for facilitating an approach to gender-based violence within the context of sexual and reproductive health care. The kit includes the following sections: Definitions; Screening Tool; Sample Stamp for Client Intake Form to Record Information on GBV; Management Checklist; Legal Framework for Service Providers Addressing GBV; Knowledge, Attitudes, and Practices Questionnaire for Health Care Providers; and Observation Guide. http://www.ippfwhr.org/whatwedo/bastatools.html

➜ **Drawing the Line: A Guide to Developing Effective Sexual Assault Prevention Programs for Middle School Students.** *American College of Obstetricians and Gynecologists, 2000.*
The document highlights components of promising programs being implemented in the United States, contains an example of the process one state chose to design and implement sexual assault prevention education programs for this age group, and includes a list of resources.
http://www.acog.com/from_home/publications/drawingtheline/index.htm

➜ **Diagnostic and Treatment Guidelines on Family Violence.**
American Medical Association, 1999.
The publication presents separate modules establishing guidelines on the following seven aspects of violence: child physical abuse and neglect and child sexual abuse; domestic violence; elder abuse and neglect; strategies for the treatment and prevention of sexual assault; mental health effects of family violence; physician guide to media violence; and a physician firearms safety guide. http://www.ama-assn.org/ama/pub/category/3548.html

➜ **Preventing Domestic Violence: Clinical Guidelines on Routine Screening.**
Family Violence Prevention Fund, 1999.
A multi-specialty, comprehensive routine screening document on domestic violence. In addition to specific guidelines for primary care, obstetrical and gynecological, family planning, urgent care, mental health, and in-patient settings, it includes an extensive bibliography, documentation forms, and other useful materials.
http://endabuse.org/programs/display.php3?DocID=31

➜ **Promoting Early and Effective Intervention to Save Women's Lives.**
Family Violence Prevention Fund, 1999.
This kit contains a series of information packets for health care providers interested in developing a comprehensive health care response to domestic violence. Packets include: General Information on the Health Care Response to Domestic Violence; The Emergency Department Response to Domestic Violence; Screening Patients for Domestic Violence; Mandatory Reporting of Domestic Violence by Health Care Providers; and Violence against People with Disabilities.
http://endabuse.org/programs/display.php3?DocID=55

➜ **Saving Women's Lives:**
Training Reproductive Health Care Providers to Address Domestic Violence in Mexico.
Family Care International, 1999.
A series of protocols to help reproductive health care workers address gender-based violence in their practices, with a specific emphasis on screening women during routine reproductive health care visits. Includes a section on working with women's groups and other NGO partners who provide social and legal support services for victims of violence.
http://www.familycareintl.org/pubs/index.html

⇝ **Say No to Violence:**
Overview of Domestic Violence and Counseling Skills Resource Handbook.
Women's Department and National Women's Commission, 1999.
This handbook produced in Belize provides a collection of strategies to aid both the
woman who finds herself in an unacceptable relationship and those who endeavor to offer
her assistance in solving her problems. The interventions that a helper can initiate are
wide-reaching but nonintrusive and are based on the belief that abused women must be
supported in finding the means of resolution that are most appropriate for each woman's
particular situations. (Not available online.)

⇝ *Violencia familiar: Enfoque desde la salud pública*
[Intra-family Violence: From a Public Health Perspective].
*Flora Tristán Center, Ministry of Health of Peru, Government of the Netherlands, Pan American Health
Organization, and World Health Organization, 1999.*
This manual outlines Peru's experiences of addressing intra-family violence from a public
health perspective. Available only in Spanish. http://www.flora.org.pe/pnuevas.htm

⇝ *¿Cómo atender a las mujeres que viven situaciones de violencia doméstica?*
Orientaciones básicas para el personal de salud
[How to Care for Women Living in Situations of Violence: Basic Orientations for
Health Personnel].
*Red de Mujeres contra la Violencia (*Network of Women against Violence*), 1998.*
The publication begins with an introduction describing what gender-based violence is, what
its different forms are and how to recognize them, GBV as a public health problem, and its
physical and psychological effects. It then presents an overview of GBV in Nicaragua, its
prevalence, and the country's response, and then concludes with a comprehensive series
of possible interventions that will help health personnel to recognize GBV and develop
effective responses. Available only in Spanish. (Not available online.)

⇝ **Intimate Partner Violence during Pregnancy: A Guide for Clinicians.**
American College of Obstetricians and Gynecologists, 1998.
Designed as a training tool for clinicians to increase understanding of the role they can play
in identifying, preventing, and reducing intimate partner violence. The slide set is designed
as an introductory or supplementary learning tool to be used in conjunction with other
reinforcing and enabling strategies, including role-playing, periodic discussions at staff
meetings, staffing changes, and institutional support. Includes a situation report and potential
areas of action for clinical staff. http://www.cdc.gov/nccdphp/drh/violence/ipvdp.htm

⇝ *Prevención de la violencia por medio de la educación en la familia y la escuela*
[Preventing Violence through Education in the Family and at School].
Corporación de Estudios de la Salud, 1998.
This document presents a training course aimed at school-aged children who demonstrate
violent tendencies and/or behavior. It proposes working with children to teach them
nonviolent conflict resolution and other coping skills. Available only in Spanish.
(Not available online.)

→ **Improving the Health Care Response to Domestic Violence: A Resource Manual for Health Care Providers.** *Family Violence Prevention Fund, 1996.*
The manual includes information to educate practitioners on screening, identification, assessment, and interventions with victims of domestic violence and their batterers; practical tools including a model hospital intervention packet outlining effective protocols and sample forms for screening, domestic violence/abuse assessment, documentation, safety planning, and discharge; and ideas to help develop and implement response strategies and programs within a variety of health care practices and settings.
http://endabuse.org/programs/display.php3?DocID=35

VI. CONVENTIONS AND DECLARATIONS

1950   Convention for the Suppression of the Traffic in Persons and of the Exploitation of the Prostitution of Others http://untreaty.un.org/English/TreatyEvent2001/pdf/19e.pdf

1974   Declaration on the Protection of Women and Children in Emergency and Armed Conflict http://heiwww.unige.ch/humanrts/instree/e3dpwcea.htm

1979   Convention on the Elimination of All Forms of Discrimination against Women http://www.un.org/womenwatch/daw/cedaw/conven.htm

1989   Convention on the Rights of the Child http://untreaty.un.org/English/TreatyEvent2001/pdf/03e.pdf

1993   World Conference on Human Rights http://www.unhchr.ch/html/menu5/wchr.htm

1993   Declaration on the Elimination of Violence against Women http://www.unhchr.ch/huridocda/huridoca.nsf/(Symbol)/A.RES.48.104.En?Opendocument

1994   Inter-American Convention on the Prevention, Punishment, and Eradication of Violence against Women (Convention of Belém do Pará) http://www.undp.org/rblac/gender/osavio.htm

1994   International Conference on Population and Development http://www.unfpa.org/icpd/background.htm

1995   Fourth World Conference on Women (Beijing) http://www.un.org/womenwatch/daw/beijing/platform/

2000   Protocol to Prevent, Suppress, and Punish Trafficking in Persons, Especially Women and Children, Supplementing the United Nations Convention against Transnational Organized Crime http://untreaty.un.org/English/TreatyEvent2001/pdf/17e.pdf

2000   United Nations' Security Council Resolution 1325 on Women, Peace, and Security http://ods-dds ny.un.org/doc/UNDOC/GEN/N00/720/18/ PDF/N0072018.pdf?OpenElement

VII. INTERNET/WEB RESOURCES

→ **Centre for Research on Violence Against Women and Children**
The Centre is one of an alliance of five research centers in Canada whose purpose is to promote the development of community-centered action research on violence against women and children and to facilitate individuals, groups, and institutions representing the diversity of the community to pursue research issues and training opportunities related to the understanding and prevention of abuse. http://www.uwo.ca/violence/index.html

✥ **Coalition against Trafficking in Women**
The Coalition is composed of regional networks and affiliated individuals and groups and serves as an umbrella that coordinates and takes direction from its regional organizations and networks in its work against sexual exploitation and in support of women's human rights. http://www.catwinternational.org/

✥ **End Violence against Women, Johns Hopkins University, Center for Communications Programs**
This site features an online collection of materials and resources on preventing violence against women. It is part of an ongoing effort to share information with health professionals who seek information and resources on this subject. http://www.endvaw.org/

✥ **End-Violence Working Group**
Sponsored by UNIFEM, this listserv unites people from over 120 countries in a virtual community that works to end violence against women. It provides information and recommendations to U.N. agencies and publications; promotes the visibility of developing country organizations working against gender-based violence; expands networking among NGO, government, international, educational, religious, and other groups; and shares information about policies, strategies, cases, and best practices. To subscribe, send an e-mail to majordomo@mail.edc.org, leave the subject line blank, and write "subscribe end-violence" in the message area. http://www.edc.org/GLG/end-violence/hypermail/

✥ **Family Violence Prevention Fund**
The Family Violence Prevention Fund, through the National Health Initiative on Domestic Violence (NHIDV), addresses the health care response to domestic violence through public policy reform and health education and prevention efforts. The NHIDV develops educational resources, training materials, and model protocols on domestic violence and screening to help health care providers better serve abused women. http://endabuse.org/

✥ **Flora Tristán Center**
Since its founding in 1979, this nongovernmental organization has worked in a number of areas to improve the living conditions of women in Peru. The Web site provides background on national and international projects and training, and contains articles and publications. (Information in Spanish only.) http://www.flora.org.pe/

✥ **Regional Training Program against Domestic Violence**
United Nations Latin American Institute for the Prevention of Crime and Treatment of the Delinquent (ILANUD)
ILANUD focuses its efforts on the sensitization and training of members of the judiciary, the penal system, ministries of health and education, and the staff of police academies and universities. (Information in Spanish only.) http://www.ilanud.or.cr/violenciadomestica

✥ **International Planned Parenthood Federation (IPPF), Western Hemisphere Region (WHR)**
The IPPF/WHR Web site contains information on its GBV projects in Latin America and the Caribbean. IPPF/WHR publishes a quarterly newsletter called *¡BASTA!*, which can be

accessed and downloaded from its Web site. *¡BASTA!* reports on the efforts of IPPF affiliates in Latin America and the Caribbean to address GBV within the framework of sexual and reproductive health and offers practical information and tools to service providers who wish to work in this area. http://www.ippfwhr.org/

❧ **Isis Internacional**
Together with the Isis affiliate offices in Manila and Kampala, Isis in Chile oversees the Program on Violence against Women, an information and communications initiative that provides informational materials and resources to organizations worldwide. (Information in Spanish only.) http://www.isis.cl/

❧ **A Life Free of Violence: It's Our Right** (United Nations Inter-Agency Campaign on Women's Human Rights in Latin America and the Caribbean)
This site is part of the UNDP's contribution to the U.N. Inter-Agency Campaign on Women's Human Rights and provides a compilation of materials provided by all partner agencies. http://www.undp.org/rblac/gender/

❧ **Minnesota Center against Violence and Abuse (MINCAVA)**
The MINCAVA Electronic Clearinghouse strives to provide a quick and easy access point to the ever-growing number of resources available online on the topic of violence and abuse. One focus of the Clearinghouse is to assist faculty and staff in developing higher education curricula on violence and abuse. The Clearinghouse shares in electronic form curricula and syllabi used in violence education programs at institutions of higher education across the United States. http://www.mincava.umn.edu

❧ **National Sexual Violence Resource Center**
A clearinghouse of information, resources, and research related to all aspects of sexual violence. Activities include collecting, reviewing, cataloguing, and disseminating information related to sexual violence; coordinating efforts with other organizations and projects; providing technical assistance and customized information packets on specific topics; and maintaining a Web site with up-to-date information. http://www.nsvrc.org

❧ **National Violence against Women Prevention Research Center (NVAWPRC)**
The Center serves as a clearinghouse for prevention strategies by keeping researchers and practitioners aware of training opportunities, policy decisions, and recent research findings. http://www.vawprevention.org

❧ **Nursing Network on Violence against Women (NNVAW)**
The NNVAW was formed to encourage the development of a nursing practice that focuses on health issues related to the effects of violence on women's lives. http://www.nnvawi.org/

❧ **Program for Appropriate Technology in Health (PATH)**
PATH is a nongovernmental organization whose mission is to improve the health of women and children. Its Web site features access to resources related to women's health and gender issues. www.path.org

➔ *Puntos de Encuentro*

Puntos de Encuentro is a nongovernmental organization in Nicaragua dedicated to communication, research, and education on issues affecting the health and development of women and adolescents. The group's Web site contains information on its programs, including *Sexto sentido*, a popular television series targeted toward adolescents which uses a gender perspective to address issues adolescents might experience in their daily lives, such as gender-based violence. (Information in Spanish only.) http://www.puntos.org.ni/

➔ **Queen Sofía Centre for the Study of Violence**

This site is a bibliographic database of Spanish and English language resources on gender-based violence/violence against women. http://www.gva.es/violencia/

➔ **Reproductive Health Outlook**

Provides links to numerous sites of organizations addressing violence against women and includes sections on gender and men and reproductive health. http://www.rho.org

➔ **Reproductive Health for Refugees Consortium (RHRC)**

This Consortium is a partnership of seven organizations dedicated to increasing access to a range of quality, voluntary reproductive health services for refugees and displaced persons around the world. Gender-based violence is one of the four essential and complementary technical areas of reproductive health on which RHRC focuses its work. The Web site also features several links to reports and guides on addressing gender-based violence in refugee settings. http://www.rhrc.org/resources/gbv/index.html

➔ **SIVIC**

This site specializes in the treatment of domestic violence and is targeted particularly toward health sector professionals. In addition to providing background information on the problem of domestic violence, the site also offers practical advice on how health care providers can identify, evaluate, and help women who are the victims of domestic violence during the course of health consultations. An initiative of the European Commission, the site contents are available in English, French, Italian, Portuguese, and Spanish. http://www.sivic.org

➔ **United Nations Development Fund for Women (UNIFEM)**

UNIFEM provides financial and technical assistance to innovative programs and strategies that promote women's human rights, political participation, and economic security. The Web site features information about international resolutions concerning violence against women, UNIFEM's work, available resources, and the application process. http://www.unifem.undp.org/trustfund/

➔ **Violence Against Women Electronic Network (VAWnet)**

Provides support for the development, implementation, and maintenance of effective violence against women intervention and prevention efforts at the national, state, and local levels through electronic communication and information dissemination. VAWnet participants, including state domestic violence and sexual assault coalitions, allied organizations, and individuals, have access to online database resources. http://www.vawnet.org

BIBLIOGRAPHY AND REFERENCES

- Campbell J. Assessing dangerousness: Violence by sexual offenders, batterers, and child abusers. Thousand Oaks, California: Sage Publications; 1995.

- Campbell J. Promise and perils of surveillance in addressing violence against women. Violence Against Women 2000;6(7):705-727.

- Claramunt C. Helping ourselves to help others. Self-care guide for those who work in the field of family violence. San José, Costa Rica: Pan American Health Organization, Women, Health, and Development Program; 1999. (Gender and Public Health Series 7).

- Claramunt C. Battered women: a working guide for crisis intervention. San José, Costa Rica: Pan American Health Organization, Women, Health, and Development Program; 1999. (Gender and Public Health Series 1).

- Claramunt C. Abuso sexual en mujeres adolescentes. San José, Costa Rica: Organización Panamericana de la Salud, Programa Mujer, Salud y Desarrollo; 2000. (Serie Género y Salud Pública 9).

- Cole P. Proceso grupal: sistematización de la experiencia de los Grupos de Ayuda Mutua (GAM). Lima, Peru: Organización Panamericana de la Salud; 1999.

- Costa Rica, Centro Nacional para el Desarrollo de la Mujer y la Familia. Plan nacional para la atención y la prevención de la violencia intrafamiliar (PLANOVI). San José, Costa Rica: Centro Nacional para el Desarrollo de la Mujer y la Familia; 1997.

- Counts D, Brown JK, Campbell JC. To have and to hit. Chicago: University of Chicago Press; 1999.

- Davidson LL, Grisso JA, García-Moreno C, García J, King VJ, Marchant S. Training programs for healthcare professionals in domestic violence [Review paper]. Journal of Women's Health & Gender-Based Medicine 2001;10(10):953.

- Edleson J. Controversy and change in batterer's programs. In: Edleson JL, Eisikovits ZC. Future interventions with battered women and their families. Thousand Oaks, California: Sage Publications; 1995:154-169.

- Ellsberg M, Claramunt C. Mid-term review of PAHO's project: Organizing and strengthening women and promoting coordinated actions between government and civil society at the local level to prevent and treat intrafamily violence against women. Managua: Pan American Health Organization; 1996.

- Ellsberg M, Clavel Arcas C. Final report. Review of PAHO's project: Towards an integrated model of care for family violence in Central America. Washington, DC: Pan American Health Organization; 2001. Available at: www.paho.org/english/hdp/hdw/lessonsfinal.PDF

- Ellsberg M, Liljestrand J, Winkvist A. The Nicaraguan network of women against violence: using research and action for change. Reprod Health Matters 1997;10:82-92.

- Ellsberg MC, Peña R, Herrera A, Liljestrand J, Winkvist A. Candies in hell: women's experiences of violence in Nicaragua. Soc Sci Med 2000; 51(11):1595-1610.

- Fawcett GM, Heise L, lsita-Espejel L, Pick S. Changing community responses to wife abuse: a research and demonstration project in Iztacalco, Mexico. Am Psychol 1999;54(1):41-49.

- Feldhaus KM, Koziol-McLain J, Amsbury HL, Norton IM, Lowestein SR, Abbott JT. Accuracy of three brief screening questions for detecting partner violence in the emergency department. JAMA 1997;277(17):1357-1361.

- García-Moreno C. Dilemmas and opportunities for an appropriate health-service response to violence against women. Lancet 2002;359:1509-1514.

- Gerbert B, Abercrombie P, Caspers N, Love C, Brostone A. How health care providers help battered women: the survivor's perspective. Women Health 1999;29(3):115-135.

- Guedes A, Bott S, Cuca Y. Integrating systematic screening for gender-based violence into sexual and reproductive health services: results of a baseline study by the International Planned Parenthood Federation, Western Hemisphere Region. Int J Gynecol Obstet 2002;78(Suppl 1):S57-S63.

- Guedes AC, Stevens L, Helzner JF, Medina S. Addressing gender violence in a reproductive and sexual health program in Venezuela. In: Haberland N, Measham D, eds. Responding to Cairo: case studies of changing practice in reproductive health and family planning. New York: Population Council; 2002.

- Gutiérrez F. La mediación pedagógica. Heredia, Costa Rica: Instituto Latinoamericano de Pedagogía de la Comunicación; 1993.

- Heise L, Ellsberg M, Gottemoeller M. Ending violence against women. Baltimore: Johns Hopkins University School of Public Health, Population Information Program; 1999. (Population Reports, Series L, 11).

- Heise L, Pitanguy J, Germain A. Violence against women: the hidden health burden. Washington, DC: World Bank; 1994. (Discussion paper 255).

- Josiah I. The health sector working with women's organizations: a case study. Proceedings of the WHO/FIGO Pre-Congress Workshop on Elimination of Violence against Women: In Search of Solutions. Copenhagen, 1998.

- Koss MP, Woodruff WJ, Koss PG. Criminal victimization among primary care medical patients: prevalence, incidence, and physician usage. Behav Sci Law 1991;9(1):85-96.

- Leye E, Githaniga A, Temmerman M. Health care strategies for combating violence against women in developing countries. Presentation at International Center for Reproductive Health, Ghent, Belgium, August 1999.

- Mandela N. World report on violence and health [Foreword]. Geneva: World Health Organization; 2002.

- McCauley J, Yurk RA, Jenckes MW, Ford DE. Inside "Pandora's box": abused women's experiences with clinicians and health services. J Gen Intern Med 1998;13:549-555.

- McFarlane J, Christoffel K, et al. Assessing for abuse: self-report versus nurse interview. Public Health Nurs 1991;8(4):245-250.

- McLeer SV, Anwar RA, Herman S, Maquiling K. Education is not enough: a system's failure in protecting battered women. Ann Emerg Med 1989;18(6):651-653.

- Motsei M. Detection of women battering in health care settings: the case of Alexandra health clinic. South Africa: Centre for Health Policy; 1993.

- Nicaragua, Ministerio de Salud. Los hombres del SILAIS Masaya: género, masculinidad y violencia intrafamiliar en las presentaciones sociales del trabajador de salud. Managua: Ministerio de Salud, Organización Panamericana de la Salud; 2001.

- Organización Panamericana de la Salud. Memoria modelos en construcción para la atención integral a la violencia intrafamiliar y el rol del sector salud. Seminario Taller Centroamericano Modelos en Construcción para la Atención Integral a la Violencia Intrafamiliar. Managua, 1997. San José, Costa Rica: OPS, Programa Mujer, Salud y Desarrollo; 1999.

- Organización Panamericana de la Salud. Redes o coaliciones de acción en violencia intrafamiliar. San José, Costa Rica: OPS, Programa Mujer, Salud y Desarrollo; 1999. (Serie Género y Salud Pública 2).

- Organización Panamericana de la Salud. Reporte comprensivo de siete investigaciones de situación de salud a nivel local según condiciones de vida con enfoque de género realizadas en Centroamérica (período 1994–1995). San José, Costa Rica: OPS, Programa Mujer, Salud y Desarrollo; 1999. (Serie Género y Salud Pública 5).

- Organización Panamericana de la Salud. Organización de redes para la prevención y atención de la violencia intrafamiliar: guía para instituciones y organizaciones comunitarias. La Paz, Bolivia: Ministerio de Salud y Previsión Social; OPS, Programa Mujer, Salud y Desarrollo; 2000.

- Organización Panamericana de la Salud. Informe del 3° Taller Centroamericano sobre el Registro, la Vigilancia y la Prevención de la Violencia Intrafamiliar y Sexual. San José, Costa Rica: OPS, Programa Mujer, Salud y Desarrollo; 2001. (Serie Género y Salud Pública 11).

- Organización Panamericana de la Salud. La planificación estratégica en las redes de lucha contra la violencia intrafamiliar en Centroamérica. San José, Costa Rica: OPS, Programa Mujer, Salud y Desarrollo; 2001. (Serie Género y Salud Pública 12).

- Organización Panamericana de la Salud. Mesa nacional para la prevención y atención de la violencia familiar: por un camino de concertación para deconstruir la violencia familiar en el Perú. Lima: OPS; 2001.

- Organization of American States. Inter-American Convention on the Prevention, Punishment, and Eradication of Violence against Women "Convention of Belém do Pará." Washington, DC: Inter-American Commission of Women; 2000. Available at: www.oas.org.

- Pan American Health Organization. Helping ourselves to help others: self-care guide for those who work in the field of family violence. San José, Costa Rica: PAHO, Women, Health, and Development Program; 2001. (Gender and Public Health Series 7).

- Pan American Health Organization. Integrated model of attention to intrafamily violence. San José, Costa Rica: PAHO, Women, Health, and Development Program; 2001. (Gender and Public Health Series 10).

- Pan American Health Organization. Research protocol: social response to family violence at the local level. San José, Costa Rica: PAHO, Women, Health, and Development Program; 2002. (Gender and Public Health Series 4).

- Parker B, Campbell J. Care of victims of abuse and violence. In: Wiscarz G, Sundeen SJ. Principles and practice of psychiatric nursing. St. Louis: Mosby; 1991.

- Quirós E. Y no viví feliz para siempre. San José, Costa Rica: Centro Nacional para el Desarrollo de la Mujer y la Familia; 1997. (Colección Metodologías. Sentir, pensar y enfrentar la violencia intrafamiliar).

- Ramellini T, Mesa S. Estrategias de intervención especializada con personas afectadas por la violencia intrafamiliar: emprendiendo un camino. San José, Costa Rica: Centro Nacional para el Desarrollo de la Mujer y la Familia; 1997. (Colección Metodologías. Sentir, pensar y enfrentar la violencia intrafamiliar).

- Red de Mujeres contra la Violencia. ¿Cómo atender a las mujeres que viven situaciones de violencia doméstica? Orientaciones básicas para el personal de salud. Managua: Red de Mujeres contra la Violencia; 1999.

- Rodríguez MA, Craig AM, Mooney DR, Bauer HM. Patient attitudes about mandatory reporting of domestic violence–implications for health care professionals. West J Med 1998;169:337-341.

- Rosales Ortiz J, Loaiza E, Primante D, Barberena A, Blandón Sequeira L, Ellsberg M. Encuesta Nicaragüense de Demografía y Salud, 1998. Managua: Instituto Nacional de Estadísticas y Censos; 1999.

- Sagot, M. La ruta crítica de las mujeres afectadas por la violencia intrafamiliar en América Latina: estudios de caso en diez países. San José, Costa Rica: Organización Panamericana de la Salud, Programa Mujer, Salud y Desarrollo; 2000.

- Shrader E, Sagot M. La ruta crítica que siguen las mujeres afectadas por la violencia intrafamiliar: protocolo de investigación. Washington, DC: Organización Panamericana de la Salud, Programa Mujer, Salud y Desarrollo; 1998.

- Shrader E, Sagot M. Domestic violence: women's way out. Washington, DC: Pan American Health Organization; 2000. (Occasional Publication 2).

- Sugg NK, Inui T. Primary care physicians' response to domestic violence: opening Pandora's box. JAMA 1992;267(23):3157-3160.

- United Nations. The Convention on the Elimination of All Forms of Discrimination against Women, 1979. Available at: www.un.org/womenwatch/daw/cedaw/frame.htm

- United Nations. Declaration on the Elimination of Violence against Women, 1993. Available at: www.unhchr.ch/huridocda/huridoca.nsf/(Symbol)/A.RES.48.104.En?Opendocument

- United Nations. Beijing Declaration and Platform for Action: Fourth Conference on Women. September 4-15, Beijing, 1995. New York: United Nations; Division for the Advancement of Women; 1995. Available at: www.un.org/womenwatch/daw/beijing/platform

- United Nations. "Let this be the reform Assembly", says Secretary-General addressing fifty-second session. New York: UN; 1997. (SG/SM/6334).
  Available at: www.un.org/News/Press/docs/1997/19970922.SGSM6334.html

- United Nations. The world's women 2000: trends and statistics. New York: UN; 2000.

- United Nations High Commissioner for Human Rights. Vienna Declaration and Programme of Action: World Conference on Human Rights. June 14-25, Vienna, 1993. Geneva: UNHCHR; 1993. Available at: www.unhchr.ch/html/menu5/wchr.htm

- United Nations Population Fund. Programme of Action: International Conference on Population and Development. September 5-13, Cairo, 1994. Available at: www.unfpa.org/icpd/background.htm

- Warshaw C, Ganley AL. Improving the health care response to domestic violence: a resource manual for health care providers. San Francisco: Family Violence Prevention Fund; 1998.

- World Health Organization. Women's health: improve our health, improve the world. WHO position paper, Fourth World Conference on Women. September 4-15, Beijing, 1995. Geneva: WHO; 1995. (WHO/FHE/95.8).

- World Health Organization. Injury surveillance guidelines. Geneva: WHO; 2001. (WHO/NMF/VIP/01.02).

- World Health Organization. The World Health Report 2001. Mental health: new understanding, new hope. Geneva: WHO; 2001.

- World Health Organization. Multi-country study on women's health and domestic violence. Geneva: WHO; 2002. (HO/FCH/GWH/02.2).

- World Health Organization. World report on violence and health. Geneva: WHO; 2002.

- Zegarra Tarqui M. Redes locales frente a la violencia familiar. Lima: Organización Panamericana de la Salud; 1999. (Serie Violencia Intrafamiliar y Salud Pública. Documento de Análisis 2).